Calming the Corona

I0115708

Calming the Corona

*Dr. Calm's Guide to Staying Strong and Finding Solace
During the Pandemic*

(Stay Calm, Think Rational, and Don't Do Anything Stupid)

The publisher is not in the business of giving medical advice. If you have any questions or concerns, please consult a physician. All work contained here is from the author's experience and research.

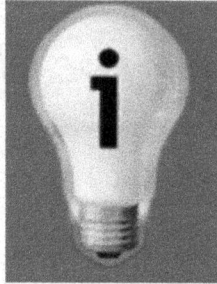

iBooks
Manhanset House
Shelter Island Hts., New York 11965-0342
Tel: 212-427-7139
bricktower@aol.com • www.ibooksinc.com
All rights reserved under the International and Pan-American Copyright Conventions. Printed in the United States by J. Boylston & Company, Publishers, New York. No part of this publication may be reproduced, stored in a retrieval system, or transmitted in any form or by any means, electronic, or otherwise, without the prior written permission of the copyright holder.
The iBooks colophon is a trademark of J. Boylston & Company, Publishers.

Library of Congress Cataloging-in-Publication Data
Dintyala, Kiran.
Calming the Corona—Dr. Calm's Guide to Staying Strong and Finding Solace During the Pandemic
p. cm.

1. HEALTH & FITNESS/Diseases/Contagious. 2. HEALTH & FITNESS/Safety.
3. MEDICAL/Health Policy.
Non-fiction, I. Title.
ISBN: 978-1-59687-895-2, Tradepaper

Copyright © 2020 by Kiran Dintyala

September 2020

Table of Contents

Acknowledgments

I am thankful to all the people involved in publishing of this book in such a short period.

First and foremost, I acknowledge the fact that I wouldn't have been able to write a single word of inspiration without the intuitive guidance provided by God and the teachings of my guru Sri Paramahansa Yogananda. Their constant presence is the guiding force of my life and an eternal source of inspiration, strength, and courage to pursue all my endeavors.

I am deeply indebted to Mr. Alan Morell, my agent and manager, who made this book possible to be published quickly.

Many thanks to Mr. John Colby, founder and the president of Brick Tower Press, for giving me an opportunity to be published by their prestigious publishing house and for being ready to work on a very tight deadline in bringing this book to life and presenting it to the world.

I appreciate very much "Chambers Group" and Timothy Troke from "FrogWater Media" for their social media and marketing expertise in building Dr. Calm brand, and I am lucky to have them in my team.

I thank Mr. Ray Bell, an Emmy award-winning producer, and a dear friend of mine, for his wisdom and advice on this journey of mine as an author and media personality, to bring my ideas to life and share my expertise with the public.

I am deeply indebted to my parents and my sister for their steadfast love and support, without which I would not have developed into the person and professional I am today.

My uncles Udaya Kumar and Murali Krishna have been of tremendous support to me and are my "go to people" for guidance during times of turmoil in my life. They have been there as strong pillars of support since my childhood, the value of which cannot be overstated.

Last but not the least, my daughter, Mayura, who gives meaning to my life and inspires me every day to progress and prosper in life, and in her beautiful ways, reminds me to live life to the fullest every moment. Without her, I am not there. Her love for me, and my love for her, is what keeps me going in life.

Preface

No one thought the coronavirus would wreak such havoc. When we saw China going through the Corona epidemic, we thought it was just a Chinese problem. Then Italy and South Korea started seeing a plethora of COVID-19 cases. Soon it spread to the United States. The virus spread quickly and became a rapidly evolving pandemic, pushing the world into panic. Thousands died. The stock market crashed, leaving investors in a state of terror. People gripped by fear and uncertainty seemed to be losing their minds. Many bought toilet paper rolls for a year, forgetting that standing in line in Costco for hours is dangerous. People stole masks from hospitals and clinics. That is what happens when we panic. We lose our rationality. Morality goes out the window. Greed and fear take over the good side of us.

On the other side, many are suffering from COVID-19 symptoms. They are afraid for themselves and their loved ones, not knowing if they will succumb to death. The fear and the anxiety are palpable across the board. Businesses have shut down. Travel plans have halted. Restaurants are not running. Schools are closed. Health care workers are scrambling, and hospital systems in coronavirus hotspots across the world are overwhelmed. And the worst of all, we don't know how long this will last. Lots of uncertainty!

We have never seen anything like this in our lifetime. The impact on the economy is huge. Both businesses and the common man are worried about their ability to survive the financial damage caused by the pandemic. Many are afraid that this may push us over into an economic recession, and the way things are going, it's already coming to be true.

More than 30 million Americans filed for unemployment insurance after the beginning of the pandemic. US GDP fell by 4.8% at an annual rate in the first quarter of 2020, the largest quarterly decline in GDP since the fourth quarter of 2008 during the global financial crisis when the US economy contracted by 8.4%. The US equities market has lost $11.5 trillion in capitalization since peaking on February 19, pushed down by coronavirus risks and a global oil-price war. The unemployment rate in the United States reached 14.7 percent in April 2020 after averaging 5.74 percent from 1948 until 2020. That's a huge jump by any standard.

So, what should we do in this circumstance? How many of us are going to die? If we survive the virus, can we survive the financial crisis? What happens if we enter a situation like the Great Depression of the 1930s? With no food to eat and no money, what happens if people start looting each other? The consequences can be terrible. People could turn to crime, drugs, domestic abuse, and suicide. We are already seeing some of that.

How do we prevent these problems? How can we weather the negative consequences of this pandemic? How can we stay calm, think rationally, and protect ourselves as well as our loved ones during these difficult times?

Using his extensive experience in the medical field, and also being a public health professional as well as an author, a speaker, and a stress management consultant, Dr. Kiran Dintyala, a.k.a. Dr. Calm, has responded quickly to this crisis and urgently written this book to help people around the globe.

Overview

This book addresses the following:

1. Why we should not panic over this pandemic.
2. How to stay sane during crisis.
3. How to recover from financial stress.
4. How to boost your immunity.
5. Why thinking rational and staying calm is the only way to overcome this pandemic.
6. How to protect yourself and your loved ones from COVID-19.
7. How to be helpful to others in a meaningful way during these difficult times.

8. What you should do during and after the pandemic to stay out of harm's way.

9. How not to lose your sleep over the coronavirus and more.

Disclaimer: This is not medical advice. This is an attempt to provide the facts available so far to the best of my knowledge. This is an attempt to provide you with the information needed to stay sane and calm during this pandemic so that you protect your mental and physical health during these difficult times.

Introduction:
Who Stole My Toilet Paper?

A few weeks ago, when I first heard that people were lining up at Costco, emptying the entire store by buying supplies for months, I couldn't believe my ears. The news of coronavirus spread like wildfire, sending the whole nation into a state of alarm. People are still terrified, not knowing what's going to happen to them next. Many died in China, Italy, and South Korea. And many are dying in the United States, Europe, and the rest of the world. What is this new virus? How dangerous is it? Is it worse than the seasonal flu? How long is it going to last? Weeks, months, even years?

Though we have learned a lot about COVID-19 the past few months, still there is a lot more to learn. We still are learning how this virus spreads and how fast it does so, how long it stays in the human body, for how long we transmit the disease to others, etc. We still are trying to understand the exact mechanism of how this virus attacks our body. We still don't have reliable data on how many people really get ill with this virus. Of those who do, how many get bad symptoms, and how many actually progress to death? Even doctors didn't know much about this virus until recently. We are learning something new about this virus every day.

As a physician, I am seeing panic all over. I am glad that the government declared this as a national emergency and sped up the process of containing this pandemic. A few weeks ago, when the World Health Organization (WHO) declared COVID-19 as a pandemic, the stock market suffered the worst crash since 1987. Many countries, including the United States, started scrambling, not knowing how to face this pandemic. Obviously, people across the world are scared too, as the virus is spreading to Central America, South America, and Africa. Things are not going to be easy for anyone.

Many are afraid that this could be the end of the world. Now, this is what happens when people are in a panic mode. In the face of uncertainty, people become irrational. Smart people start doing stupid things. They will be overcome by their emotions. The end result is something like what we were seeing in Costco. For example, people started buying all the toilet paper from Costco and other stores, six to ninth months' supply. The same is true for many other products and supplies. But they were not realizing the dangers of standing in line at Costco without a mask, which few wore back in March. Some may actually have contracted the virus, gotten sick, and died because of that. Lack of toilet paper for the next six months will not kill them but getting exposed to huge crowds at Costco can certainly do so.

At the beginning of this pandemic, I went to Costco to buy a few groceries and I had to turn back because it was packed. And I saw many people were not wearing masks. Maybe it's because they couldn't find any masks. Even some hospitals were and still are in shortage of masks. It's because of over-consumption. Many started using our resources injudiciously, triggered by fear. For example, one of the hospitals I know mandated all their employees to wear a mask all the time and they had to change their mask every four hours. At that rate, I could tell that they would run out of their masks in a short period of time. Then, when they actually required masks, they were not able to find them.

I also saw that people were stealing masks from hospitals and urgent care centers. People lose their rationality and morality when they panic. The same is true with hand sanitizers. Almost all stores that I know ran out of them overnight. If you saw on the news, a greedy man bought 17,700 bottles of hand sanitizer in Tennessee to resell and profit from them, taking advantage of this pandemic. That's insane!

If a small section of the population uses most of the community's resources or misuses them, what's going to happen to the rest? If your child has three months of formula or baby food but because of that your neigh-bors' and many other children have nothing to eat or drink for days to weeks, what's going to happen? Is it going to lead to a civil war? Will people start stealing from each other? We need to think about these things before we act in panic. I personally have not stocked up on anything. I have stuff available at home for only two weeks at the beginning of this pandemic, and I am taking one step at a time, buying only small quantities, being mindful of others' needs.

I am confident that we are going to survive this pandemic. I believe there are enough good people in the world, in the government, and in the health care system and we will find solutions to survive this pandemic. *Whether we do that gracefully or not depends on whether we stay calm or not.* I can guarantee that as a nation, as a community, as a family, and as an individual, if we remain calm and think rationally, we have better chances to emerge out of this crisis minimally harmed. On the contrary, if our actions are driven by rabid fear, we are sure to succumb to bad consequences. We all have to face this challenge together. We need to use our resources judiciously and be sensible in our decision-making.

Just for example, let me give you an alternative situation where people are not in a panic mode—they are sensible and are taking good precautions like handwashing and wearing masks as needed. They are going about their routine normally but avoiding crowds. No one is gathering in large numbers in parks, on beaches, or in-house parties. People are all peacefully buying what they want for the next few days to weeks. No one is overconsuming. We all will have toilet paper without standing in line for hours. Our children will have food to eat as usual. We go about our life as peacefully as we can, given the situation. This is a completely different scenario. Don't you think we are going to be better in this scenario rather than being in a panic mode?

So, how do we do that? How do we create this alternative scenario where people are calm and rational? That's what this book is about. To get to that, we need to learn certain facts about this viral illness, and we need to practice simple things that bring us calm. It's not complex. It just requires a little patience and open-mindedness to learn and implement a few simple disciplines. Let's do that now before it's too late!

Chapter 1:
The Doctor's Advice

As a doctor, my first priority is your health and well-being. So, let's start off with important precautions we all must take based on the research facts available to date:

1. **First things first:**
    i. Take necessary precautions as outlined by your health care and government officials.
    ii. When in doubt, it's better to be overcautious than to be undercautious.
    iii. Be rational in your thinking and judicious in your actions.

2. **Here are some safety tips:**
    i. Avoid crowds or any large gatherings.
    ii. Avoid close contact with people who are sick (especially those who have cold like symptoms).
    iii. Use hand sanitizer or wash your hands often with soap and water for at least 20 seconds.
    iv. Avoid touching your eyes, nose, and mouth with unwashed hands.
    v. Clean and disinfect frequently touched objects and surfaces.
    vi. Take personal responsibility to get tested or stay isolated if you feel sick or get exposed to sick people. Stay home if you are sick but your symptoms are mild (mild cough, mild fevers, no chest pain or difficulty in breathing, mild diarrhea). Self-quarantine for at least 14 days.

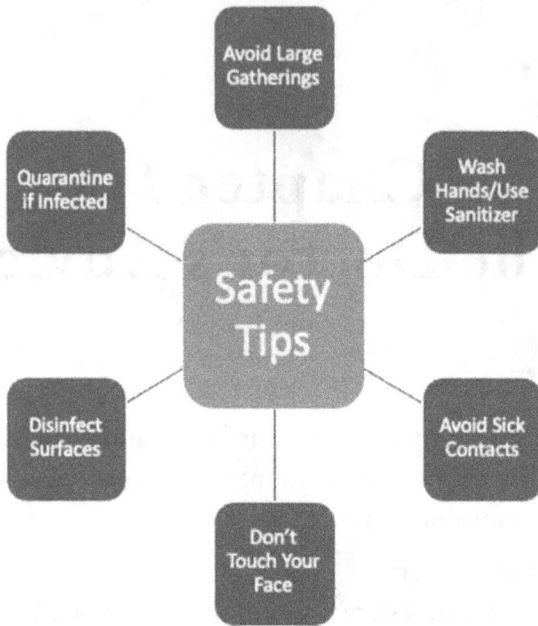

Figure 1

vii. Call your doctor or go to the hospital if your symptoms are getting severe (high fever, persistent cough and phlegm, severe diarrhea, difficulty in breathing, severe chest pain, severe headaches, severe tiredness, etc.)

3. **Know these facts to alleviate your anxiety:**
   i. Remember that this is not the end of the world.
   ii. As per the World Health Organization (WHO) report from the initial sample of 44,500 confirmed cases in Wuhan, China:
      a. The majority of infected people have an uncomplicated or mild illness (81%).
      b. Some will develop severe illness requiring oxygen therapy (14%).
      c. Only 5% will develop critical illness.
      d. Remember, the data is evolving. These are only numbers from those who were tested. Lot of people are probably not tested and had milder illness with no symptoms, thus escaping from the statistics. If we take that into

consideration, the percentage of people who get critically ill is possibly lower than being reported.

iii. So, don't imagine the worst. Stay positive. Take precautions but do not panic.

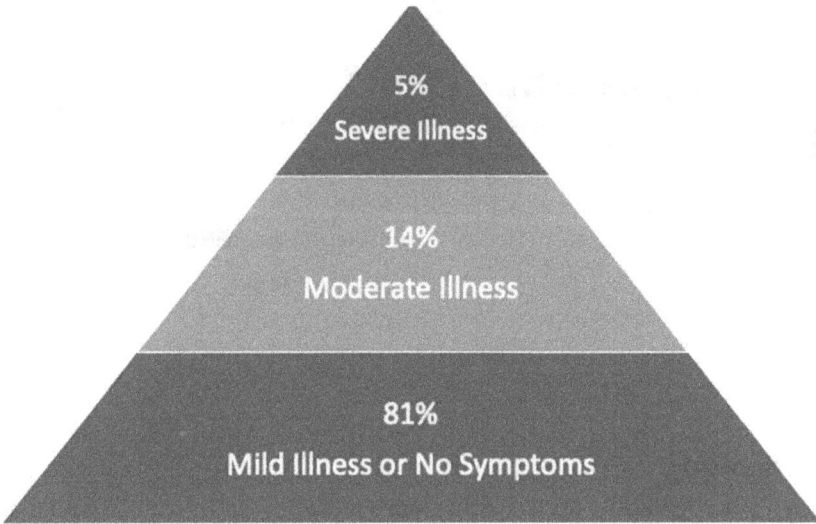

5%
Severe Illness

14%
Moderate Illness

81%
Mild Illness or No Symptoms

Figure 2

4. **If you are elderly and have preexisting conditions, take extra precaution.**

i. People with preexisting illnesses and the older population are at a higher risk to progress to critical illness.

  a. If you have a preexisting lung disease like asthma or COPD, you have to be extra careful.

  b. The same is true if you have diabetes, cancer, or other diseases that impair your immunity.

  c. If you are above age 60, especially above 80, do all that you need to stay away from the virus. Take extreme precaution.

ii. **If you are young, you may not have symptoms even when you are infected.** However, being young doesn't completely protect you either. Do not disregard the precautions because you feel all right. You have a high chance to spread the disease to others. You may be responsible for the death of your friend or family member if you don't take precautions. You don't want that burden on you. Be wise. Be smart in your decisions.

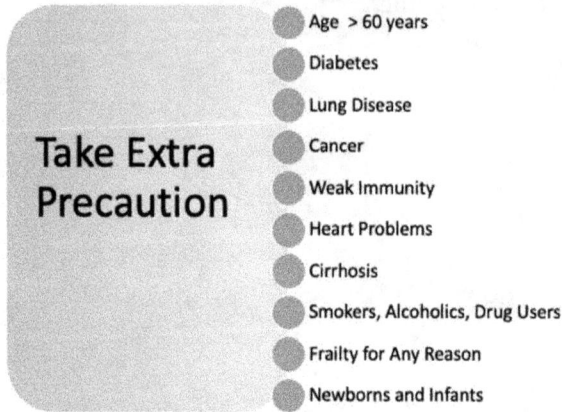

Take Extra Precaution

- Age > 60 years
- Diabetes
- Lung Disease
- Cancer
- Weak Immunity
- Heart Problems
- Cirrhosis
- Smokers, Alcoholics, Drug Users
- Frailty for Any Reason
- Newborns and Infants

Figure 3

5. **Stay calm**
   i.   We know for a fact that stress reduces your immunity and makes you susceptible to the common cold and other infections.
   ii. That is true for coronavirus SARS-CoV-2 also.
   iii. Your greatest protector is your immunity.
   iv. Avoid stress and protect your immunity.
   v.   Staying calm and eating nutritious food boosts your immunity.
   vi. So, eat well, sleep well, and exercise well.
   vii. Relax your mind.

It is imperative that we take precaution because we cannot help but notice the havoc being created by the coronavirus pandemic. This is nothing like what we've seen in our lifetime. The last major pandemic that affected millions of people and created such a massive impact on human life is the Spanish flu of 1918, which infected 500 million people. That was one-quarter of the world population at that time. It led to an estimated 50–100 million deaths. Around the same time, World War I killed 50 million people. A couple of decades later, World War II consumed another 75 million people. Those are the three major catastrophes in the past 100 years.

The reason for sharing this information is to impress upon you the seriousness of the disease we are facing. *It's important to acknowledge the reality we are seeing because that's the only way to appropriately respond to and overcome this challenge.* If we are afraid of the reality and do not acknowledge it, that's equivalent to being delusional. *As long as we are delusional, we will not overcome the problems we face.* Some people are simply saying that this is like flu and people are overreacting. That's not true. So far, based on what we know about this virus, it spreads faster than flu. It's possibly more virulent than flu but we don't know that for sure. Virulence is a term used to describe how dangerous the virus is. Also, *we as a community lack herd immunity, which makes it more dangerous than flu.* Herd immunity is the resistance to the spread of a contagious disease within a population because of a high proportion of individuals who are immune to the disease, especially through vaccination.

Because flu has been around for some time, we know a whole lot more about flu than the novel coronavirus. We know how flu spreads, we have a vaccine, and we have a medication (Tamiflu) to treat flu. The challenge with coronavirus is that we don't know exactly how it spreads. We are still trying to figure that out. We don't know how long it stays in the air. We currently believe it may stay in the air for 3–4 hours as aerosols. Also, it stays on cardboard for 24 hours and plastic and steel up to 72 hours, according to emerging research. Still, there are a lot of unknowns. *When we are facing the unknown it's better to be safe than sorry.* This is especially true when we know that people are really getting sick and dying.

The number of deaths due to coronavirus as of today, May 16, is around 311,425. It has infected more than 4.6 million people so far around the globe. In the United States, it's estimated that 100,000–200,000 deaths could be the best-case scenario. As of today, we are at 88,730 deaths. That's much worse than flu, which typically kills 30,000–60,000 people per year in the U.S. The frightening thing is the complete unpreparedness and lack of resources to face the COVID-19 pandemic in its early stages, resulting in a huge death toll. Because of the mass panic, there was injudicious overuse of our resources, leaving us all scrambling for PPE (personal protective equipment), especially the health care professionals at the frontline. ***If doctors and nurses are not protected, there won't be anyone to protect you and your loved ones.*** Fortunately, after eight weeks into the pandemic, we are definitely better prepared. But the pandemic is far from over. With the reopening of the economy and some people failing to take precautions, we could see a rapid surge in the number of COVID cases. Beware! The danger has not passed yet.

Chapter 2:
Overcoming the Panic of the Pandemic

As a physician, I get so many phone calls from my family and friends seeking advice regarding COVID issues. Also, I see patients and their family members totally unnerved every day. First of all, let me say that I understand your anxiety during these challenging times. I truly do. But we need to find a way to overcome these negative emotions for our own good. *Adding panic to the pandemic is like adding gasoline to the wildfire.* The spread of disease is already fast and devastating enough and we don't need to make it worse. *Apart from the physical illness, what makes it even worse is the public panic. If we all become fear-stricken, we will be our worst enemies, even more than the virus.* Stress degrades your immunity and makes you more susceptible to infections. That's the last thing we want because immunity is our greatest protector from this virus. We must protect it by all means. So, we have to find a way to calm ourselves and handle this gracefully.

To say not to worry and everything will be all right in the midst of a pandemic when thousands of people are dying is false assurance. It's dishonest advice and I am not going to do that. Rather, *I am going to prepare you to face the pandemic by helping you stay strong and calm in the midst of the chaos that we are seeing.* That's the only true way to overcome this pandemic and come out of it least harmed.

There are three ways to overcome fear and anxiety during these difficult times. Let's look at each, one by one.

Overcome the Panic of the Pandemic

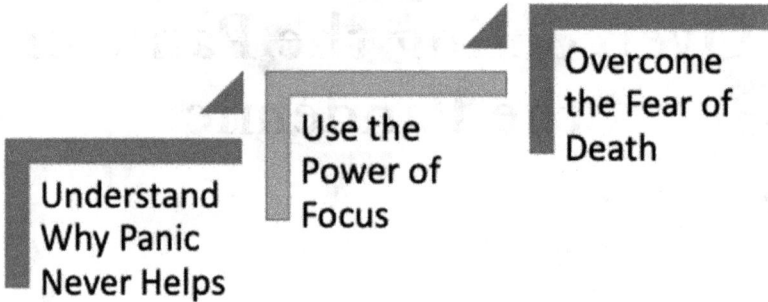

Overcome the Fear of Death

Use the Power of Focus

Understand Why Panic Never Helps

Figure 4

1. **Understand why panic never helps and why actually it is detrimental to you.**
    i. It doesn't matter what your situation is, panic actually worsens it. For example, if someone is bitten by a snake, if they panic and run around, the poison is going to spread faster and kill that person. So, the right thing to do here is stay calm, think rationally, apply a tourniquet, call for help, and take the poison out. Similarly, you just getting afraid of the coronavirus is not going to help. Take precaution. That helps.
    ii. Despite taking precaution, if you get exposed to the *novel coronavirus*, do not panic. Studies show that a majority of people do well even if they get infected. 81% will have no or mild symptoms. 14% will have severe symptoms but recover soon.
    iii. So, the chances are much higher for you to do well than getting really sick. So, ***do not imagine a fearful future. It's not worth living in fear constantly, and the worst possible future you are imagining may never come to pass.***
    iv. If it does happen that you or your loved gets critically ill, there is little you can do about it. Then why fear? Fear doesn't serve

you in this situation. Do your best to remain calm and follow the instructions given by your doctors.

v. The expected number of deaths in the United States as predicted by experts is 100,000–200,000. That means the rest of the population, more than 329 million people, are going to do well, right? Isn't that amazing?

2. **Understand the power of focus. Whatever you focus on appears real to you.**

   i. *We need to start focusing on the positive side of the pandemic* or else we all are going to die of panic before the pandemic passes. Let us stay optimistic. *The beautiful thing is that our reality changes based on the information we focus upon.* We have that power within us and it's time we use it to our benefit. So, how do we do that?

   ii. *First, stop consuming negative information.* Constantly focusing on bad news is only going to make you feel anxious and worried. Ration the amount of news you watch. Possibly, spend just 20 minutes in the morning and 20 minutes in the evening to get all the information that you need.

   iii. *Avoid the social media frenzy.* Avoid inflammatory posts. Don't get dragged into pessimistic discussions. Stay positive. Discuss good things that uplift you and others. Share success stories that give hope to others.

   iv. *Choose reliable sources of information.* When there is uncertainty, it is hard to differentiate fact from fake news. Seek trustworthy sources like the World Health Organization (WHO), Centers for Disease Control and Prevention (CDC), Johns Hopkins Coronavirus Resource Center, or some other source you are familiar with and that you trust.

   v. *Take one day at a time.* This world is not coming to an end because of COVID-19. So stay strong. Stay hopeful. After this pandemic this over, you'll be thinking, "Is that all? Why did I panic? If I knew I would be all right, I wouldn't have panicked!"

   vi. ***Enjoy the free time at hand.*** Watch feel-good movies. Play games with friends and family. Read something inspiring. Distract your mind. Do something productive.

   vii. ***Practice relaxation exercises.*** Relaxing your mind and body helps you feel better and boost your immunity. A calm mind will give you the strength needed to stay rational and fight this pandemic.

3. Overcome the fear of death

   i. All the panic that we are seeing in the world is because of the fear of death. But why should we fear death? ***Those who are afraid of death die every day in their mind,*** paralyzed by fear, anxiety, and panic. But ***those who are courageous only die once.*** Decide who you want to be.

   ii. For ***the wise, death is nothing but the next journey in life.*** No need to be afraid of death. Those who are dead are at peace. It is the living who suffer the most.

   iii. Once we overcome the fear of death, the panic and the parade of craziness will stop. Things can be done in a more orderly fashion.

   iv. ***We need to act like soldiers in the battlefield*** now, to fight this deadly pandemic. We are not going to win if we sulk in sorrow. We will definitely win if we stay strong, stay calm, and think rationally.

   v. ***Let us not be paralyzed by fear but let us paralyze the pandemic*** by thinking logically and taking necessary precaution. If we do so, a vast majority of us will do well and survive this pandemic.

   vi. Remember, we are not human beings with a soul. We are spiritual beings with a human body. ***Let's sing the songs of courage to our souls and strengthen our mind with positive thoughts.***

   vii. I am sure this shall pass, and we shall live on.

Chapter 3:
Iron Man Saves the Planet Again—This Time from COVID

I am writing this in the midst of the COVID pandemic as thousands of people are dying each day. As each week is passing by, the way I am writing this book is evolving. As a doctor, I see many of my colleagues reporting a vast number of patients coming to the hospitals every day feeling sick, requiring ventilator support, and fighting death in the ICU. I have never seen or heard anything of this sort so far in my life. My colleagues haven't either. Yes, it's frightening. Yes, it's demoralizing. Yes, it's insane. But we need to stay sane to fight this pandemic. We need to stay strong to withstand the incoming. For that, we need to stay calm and clearheaded. That's the only way we will be able to think rationally, make smart decisions, and be a formidable opponent to the Corona Demon.

We cannot be overtaken by fear. We cannot succumb to doomsday theories. **The world is not coming to an end.** We need to keep focusing on the good that is still happening in the world. We need to maintain an optimistic view of this world. You may be thinking: How is that possible? Yes, it is possible. Look around you. Look at the statistics. A vast majority of people are recovering from this disease.

Statistics show that 81% have mild or no symptoms; 14% have severe symptoms but recover without any long-term consequences; 5%

will have critical illness. So far, 88,000 people have died in the US. Yes, that's a significant number of people dying, but still a vast majority of people—greater than 95% or even 98% of people—are surviving the pandemic.

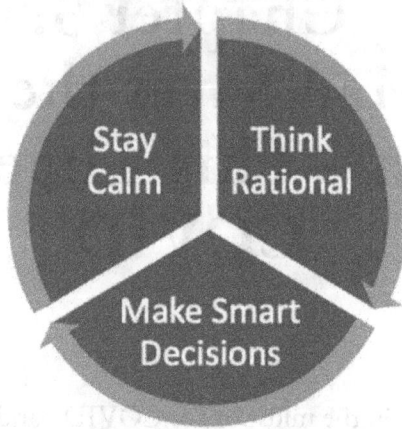

Be an Iron Man with Strong Will

Figure 5

If we dig deeper into statistics, I can confidently say that the death rate is much less than what is actually being reported. This is because you need to differentiate CFR (case fatality rate) from IFR (infection fatality rate). The difference is, in CFR you calculate deaths based on the number of people who died among the confirmed cases. But the truth in situations like this pandemic is, there are so many more unconfirmed cases, most likely because they are mildly ill. If you take all of them into account, and then calculate the number of deaths, you will get IFR. That's the real number you are looking for and that is not what is reported by media typically. Also, it is hard for us to know the real number of infected people as we are still in the middle of the pandemic and we still haven't tested people rigorously.

I will share with you the latest data from New York City, the epicenter of COVID in the United States, as analyzed by Worldometer based on the data provided by New York City, the New York State antibody study, and the excess deaths analysis by the CDC. Click the link below for more details: https://www.worldometers.info/coronavirus/coronavirus-death-rate/)

As of May 1:

1. The actual cases are 1.7 million, 10 times the number of confirmed cases.
2. Actual deaths are 23,000, almost twice the number of confirmed deaths.
3. Infection Fatality Rate is 23k/1.7M = 1.4% IFR. That means 98.6% of people who are infected recover.
4. Crude Mortality Rate (CMR) is 23k/8.4M = 0.28%. Out of a total population of 8,398,748 in New York City, 23,430 died, which is 280 deaths per 100,000 population, or 1 death for every 358 people.
5. The New York City infection rate and deaths are going to be worse than the average city in America, where it is less populated. But, even in New York City, > 98.6% are doing well.

The harsh truth is that we won't be able to save all the people on this earth. Unfortunately, some will die. We need to accept this fact, whether we like it or not. Yes, it's difficult but we have no choice. This pertains to me, you, and all of us. But, as you see from the numbers, most people will come out all right from this pandemic.

Recently, I received a call from my mother saying she got a sore throat that started a couple of days ago. I have a cousin who has a fever of 100 whom I spoke with him this morning. He was literally panicking. My daughter, whom I love the most, has been coughing for the past few days. You see, many of my family members are in a situation that's concerning. I myself recovered from a bout of illness recently. *Now, I have a choice—panic or stay calm. I'd rather choose the latter.*

I know by experience that if I panic, it's not going to help me or my loved ones. Then why should I panic? I will panic when I am on a ventilator. Even then, I know for a fact that panicking is not going to help. As a doctor, I know that people who have high anxiety have a difficult time on ventilators, requiring higher doses of sedation and a greater risk of complications. So, the truth is, the only logically appealing and helpful choice we have is to stay calm and fight hard.

We must stay strong like an IRON MAN, not so much in our physical makeup but in our mental temperament. We must be determined to be tough in the midst of this challenge. We must strongly will ourselves to stay healthy. ***This stuff is beyond your body. It's mind over body.*** We must strongly suggest to ourselves that we will be all right. Let's use our minds to boost our immunity, our greatest weapon to fight the coronavirus. This I learned from my dad from a young age. As far as I remember, he never let the thought of illness come near him. So, he rarely became ill. Even when he was ill, he never entertained the thought of feeling sick. He continued to carry on with his duties, as if nothing had happened. Yes, he rested, but he didn't complain. He didn't display signs of weakness either in his demeanor or in his words. That quality in me, I got from him. I am glad to say that in the past thirty years, I got sick only once. Prior to that, the last time I was sick was when I was a fifth-grader, due to typhoid. That's it! So, a strong mind definitely helps fight this demon of corona, which is gripping the whole world in fear.

We need to become iron men and women with iron minds to put this pandemic in iron cuffs. No Marvel's Avenger is going to come to save you. You need to become one. Stay safe, take precaution, and be strong! That's my message. ***If we remain tough and weather the situation, we can again reclaim all that we have lost materially. Remember, you are the true treasure, not the material possessions you accumulated.*** And we all have the ability to tap into our inner strength, our inner resilience, which is waiting to be awakened. It's time to ***awaken the IRON MAN within.***

Every single person has an important role to play in this endeavor. If you determine to be strong, it will help not only you but many around you. You will be the inspiration for many looking up to you. ***But staying strong doesn't mean that you become cocky*** and go out and infect people. Stay home. Stay disciplined. Stay positive. Stay calm. Be mentally tough. That's what staying strong means in this context. Let's do that now! That's how we save ourselves, our family, and our planet!

Some of you may be thinking: Just because I determine to be strong, would it really help prevent the infection? That's a good question. What I noticed in my experience as a doctor, having seen thousands of patients, is that when a person is mentally strong, he often does well physically too. I have so many instances when my patients have to go for medical procedures and the ones who are anxious to begin with end up getting unexpected complications or endure a prolonged recovery, and those who are strong mentally tend to come out least harmed even when they undergo complicated procedures.[1]

This doesn't mean that mental strength alone is going to protect you from all the diseases in this world. There are many factors that determine our health: Our genetics, the weather, our environment, the bacteria and viruses around, lifestyle, nutrition, the stress in life, and so on. All these factors directly or indirectly influence our health and well-being. Though some factors like genetics and weather are beyond our control, there are many under our control. We can choose our mindset, what we eat, our life-style, and to some extent our environment.

A man with an iron mind and unflinching determination turns the odds in his favor and achieves what he wants in life. Let me give you a real-life example: Diabetes runs in our family. My grandmother, my father, my two aunts, my three cousins, and many other family members have been diagnosed with diabetes. But *one of my uncles turned the tide by strongly determining himself not to have diabetes.* I remember from a young age that he used to be very attentive in protecting his physical health. He used to run for miles every day and he still continues that today even after 25 years of that initial determination. He is not a man with lots of free time on his hands. As an engineer and a top business executive, he is busy and also has difficult personal responsibilities. Yet he made time to take care of his health and reversed the genetics of diabetes in his favor. That's the kind of will I am talking about, which inspires us to take action to keep us healthy and strong. The same mindset will also help you fight this pandemic by doing the right things necessary to safeguard yourself from the infection and endure the difficult times we are going through.

---

[1] Preoperative Anxiety as a Predictor of Mortality and Major Morbidity in Patients >70 Years of Age Undergoing Cardiac Surgery, https://www.ncbi.nlm.nih.gov/pmc/articles/PMC3677723/

Chapter 4:
Four Forces That Pull You Out of Despair

"Thomas Schaefer, the finance minister of Germany's Hesse state, has committed suicide apparently after becoming 'deeply worried' over how to cope with the economic fallout from the coronavirus, state premier Volker Bouffier said on Sunday," **reported the TRT news outlet.**

He left behind a wife and two beautiful children in sorrow. That's terrible news.

"A man suspected to be infected with Covid-19 allegedly committed suicide by jumping off the seventh floor of a Safdarjung Hospital building," **reported the *Economic Times of India*.**

"Some areas of the country see an increase in suicide related-calls as coronavirus spreads" **reported the *Sacramento Bee*.**

"Top E.R. Doctor Who Treated Virus Patients Dies by Suicide," **reported the *New York Times*.**

"She tried to do her job, and it killed her," said the father of Dr. Lorna M. Breen, who worked at a Manhattan hospital hit hard by the coronavirus outbreak.

When I read these news articles, I was distraught. ***How dire a person's situation must have been if they thought suicide was the only way out of their problems.*** My deepest condolences to their families and loved ones.

What should we do to stop further suicides? We are living indeed in desperate times. ***The truth is, when dealing with a virus for which we have no cure or treatment, our chances to win are low if we just depend on our physical resources.*** We need to unleash our mental and spiritual potential to face such crises. Yes, the health care personnel are doing their best, but they can only do so much. We only have limited resources. ***While the physically sick are being treated in the hospitals, we need to find a way to protect the mental health of the population from the coronavirus crisis.*** That's pivotal for our success with the COVID pandemic.

If we can help people remain strong and stay hopeful, they will find innovative ways to bounce back from this pandemic and regain their overall well-being, whether it's physical, financial, or social. I am sure the governments will help resurrect and rebuild our economic systems. We will rise again to be prosperous. We will thrive. ***We as human beings have survived many atrocities, including the world wars. History is proof that we human beings are resilient beings. We will survive this pandemic too.***

There are four forces that help us dispel despair and come out strong in the face of adversity. Here they are:

1. **Hope:** In the midst of gloom and doom, the most important thing people need is hope. ***When people lose hope, they've already lost half the battle. When they find hope, they find every-thing else needed to win. So, never lose hope.*** Time and again in my life I noticed that when I lost hope, I found myself in deep trouble. When I had hope, I somehow figured out the solution for my problems, no matter how dire my situation was. This happened so many times in my life, whether it was a financial crisis, a relation-ship breakdown, career upheaval, the loss of a loved one, or some-thing else, that I do not doubt anymore the ***"power of hope." One experience after another taught me that there is always light at the end of the tunnel.*** We need to keep believing in it and keep moving forward. All of a sudden, you will find the effulgence of light that dispels the darkness of despair. You will find solutions to your problems.

The Four Forces That Dispel Despair

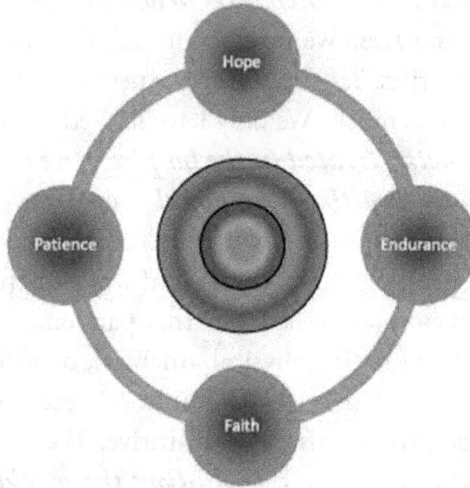

Figure 6

2. **Faith:** As you move forward with hope in life, your faith will be tested. During those times, whether you come out of the adversity or not depends on whether you use the power of faith or not. ***Faith is essentially your belief in something greater than you.*** In situations like COVID, where none of the doctors and scientists have answers for us yet, we need to believe in something, whether it is God, a Higher Power, the Universe, your Higher Self, or something else that you believe is going to help you through the situation. ***If you look at human history, it has been proven multiple times that faith can move mountains.*** I don't literally mean moving mountains, but faith can definitely help us overcome mountainous challenges. You don't have to go back to the story of David and Goliath for that. You can find that in Serena Williams, where she consistently aced the game, overcoming mammoth challenges. She proved herself a champion again and again, despite many hurdles. Serena's faith is like a secret weapon, a stealthy supply of strength and perseverance that some observers say is as vital to her game as her 120 mph serve. So, if you hold on strongly to your faith, it will help you through these difficult times.

3. **Patience:** No matter how smart, strong, and skilled you are, you will fail in life if you are not patient enough. ***Patience is a virtue. Those who have patience will beat all the odds to achieve their goals in life.*** Their dreams will come true sooner or later because of their patience. With the current situation with COVID and home isolation, a lot of people are losing their patience. I will talk about my own family first. My dad is very frustrated now, not knowing what to do at home during home isolation. He is used to going out and spending time with friends for many hours each day. Now he can't. I advise that we all remain calm and patient during home isolation. It's not the worst thing in the world. If you understand that being home is much better than being at the frontline like health workers risking their lives, it will change your perspective. Enjoy your time off during home isolation. Consider it an unexpected vacation, a virtual one where you explore the world from home. Distract yourself with some kind of work or hobby. Watch movies. Reconnect with your family and friends. Read books. Play board games at home. There are so many things one can do to remain sane and patient during this home isolation.

4. **Endurance:** Life is a marathon. Not a sprint. There are times even when you have high hopes, strong faith, and have remained patient, you still may not reach your goals. You still may not come out of the tunnel of despair. It's because there is another factor that's vital but is not exercised by most people. That's endurance. I also call it resilience. We all are born with that resilience and it gives us the ability to be flexible and adapt to challenges. It gives us the strength to withstand the greatest vicissitudes of life. As a physician I have seen cancer patients and people with severe problems bounce back again and again, beating all odds, when least expected. ***Human spirit is unbreakable. Use it to your advantage now.*** Do not give in to the negativity around you. Lift your spirits up. ***Smile through the problems like nothing happened. Everyone can smile when things are going well. Only a "hero" can smile when surrounded by difficulties. Be the hero of your life.*** Keep moving forward. I am sure you will be all right. I am sure you will come out of this unharmed and untainted at your core.

Chapter 5:
Finding Peace During Times of Crisis

A time comes in everyone's life when all that we have will be lost and our happiness will be threatened from all directions. It could be the loss of a loved one, material possessions, relationships, money, and career, or something else that we hold dear to our heart. During those times, no words can do justice to the pain that people go through. It's no easy task to bring solace to them despite the ceaseless attempts by friends and family to counsel them.

I know it because I have been there. During those times, I found great relief through powerful teachings that I accidentally stumbled upon. Those, I am going to share with you. As a physician, I had the privilege to share these teachings and have seen tremendous positive change in people's lives. This is regardless of their color, race, economic status, age, country of origin, or any other variable. *All you have to do is wholeheartedly apply these teachings.*

The Foundation of Peace and Joy

There are two powerful pillars that act as the foundation of peace and joy in our lives. They are *Innate Health* and *Resiliency*.

Innate Health is your natural state of mental well-being where your happiness is not dependent on external conditions. We all are born with it. No exceptions. To be peaceful and joyful is our true nature. If we observe little children, this truth will be evident.

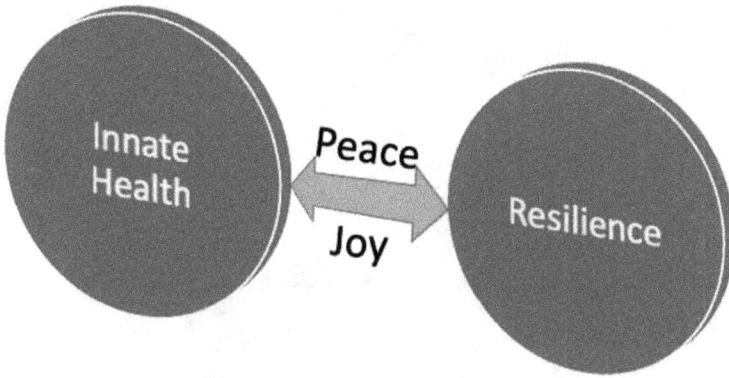

Figure 7

They are naturally happy. They don't have to read books, they don't have to attend seminars, and they don't even have to meditate. How is that possible? The only explanation is that we are born that way.

However, as we become adults, we slowly condition our happiness to various things. Initially, it is a toy, then a bike, and later a car, home, money, career, perfect relationship, or something else. Soon, *we become dependent on external factors to derive our happiness. That's called conditional happiness.* When these external conditions are threatened—for example, loss of job, loss of money, loss of loved ones, loss of relationships, etc.—we feel distressed. This is the horrible situation many are experiencing during this pandemic, and too many of these unfortunate events are happening at once.

To feel unhappy during such loss is only natural and is understandable. That's part of being human. *But we humans tend to brood over our losses for an extended period of time. That we must avoid or else we will end up getting depressed.* So, how do we avoid that? How do we pull ourselves out of these painful emotions?

The first thing to realize is, what we have lost in these situations is our conditional happiness, not our unconditional happiness. *Our true happiness—i.e., our unconditional happiness, our innate health— is still intact within, waiting to be tapped into.* During these difficult times, if you could access your innate health, you will find the solace you are looking for.

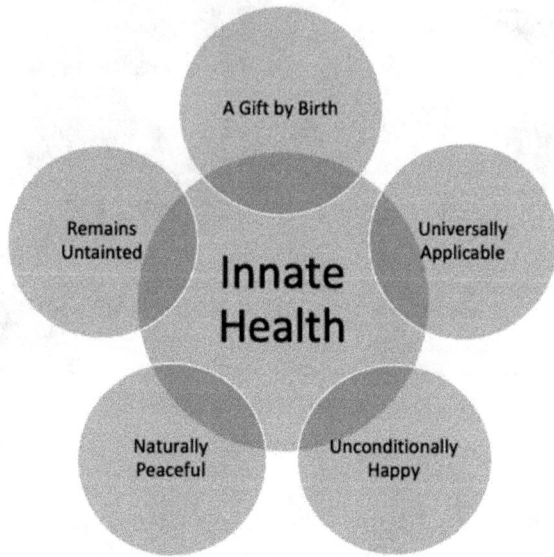

Figure 8

That is what happened to me many years ago when my career was in jeopardy, when I was in a major financial crisis, when I lost a loved one, when my relationship broke apart, and when the health of my family members was threatened. Time and again, my innate health came to my rescue. I was able to find peace no matter how dire my situation was.

Your innate health, the peace within, is like an ocean. It's vast and inexhaustible. The situations we face in life are like the waves of the ocean. They come and go. If you identify yourself with the waves, you will feel frightened. If you identify yourself with the ocean, you will be at peace. Even if there are giant waves of tumult at the surface, right beneath those waves, the ocean is still plain and peaceful. Our mind is the same. It's like an ocean.

The life circumstances we face can be compared to the waves happening at the surface. Deep within, you are a peaceful being. If you focus too much on the waves of life circumstances, you will be pulled into them and get thrashed and flailed around. We need to ride these waves gracefully and get to the place where the ocean is peaceful. That is the only sure-shot way to find peace during times of tumult.

The good news is that ocean of peace is waiting for you within. Your journey toward that peace must start now!

The easiest way to tap into that peace is letting your thoughts settle and seeing that eternal peace behind them. There are many ways to experience that. Meditation is one way. Understanding thoughts and how they affect us is another way. We will discuss both in this book as we move forward.

The deeper we enter this ocean of peace, the harder it will be for the waves of external situations to affect us. That's the state of mind we all need to achieve. And there is no time better than now to do that. *It is during the times of crisis that we must rise up to the challenge, lest we sink deeper into the pit of misery.*

Necessity is the mother of motivation. Use these challenging times to inspire you to learn this new way of living and prepare yourself for the next catastrophe, so that you can remain unshakable amid crashing worlds. Even if you are not directly affected by this pandemic, I strongly urge you to adopt this style of simple living where you can be happy regardless of external conditions. *Who knows what catastrophic event is going to visit you in the future? You better get yourself ready for that now.*

Now, let's discuss **Resilience**, the second pillar that helps you build a lasting foundation of peace and joy.

Life happens. No matter how prepared we are, there would be things that we will never be able to predict and never be ready to face. Let's accept that fact. Otherwise, we would get stuck in those situations, blaming ourselves, thinking this should have never happened, how terrible things are, and we should've never been in that situation, etc. This *self-blaming continues forever unless we accept things for what they are.* Once you accept, it eases a lot of pressure on you, and you can get yourself ready to bounce back from those difficult circumstances.

Resilience is your innate capacity to bounce back from difficult life situations, no matter how catastrophic they are. Yes, when we are going through troubles, they appear insurmountable, but we can overcome them if we don't give up, if we remain calm, and keep looking for solutions. This I have found to be true again and again in my life, no matter what the situation is. *I am an ordinary man. If I can do it, you can too.*

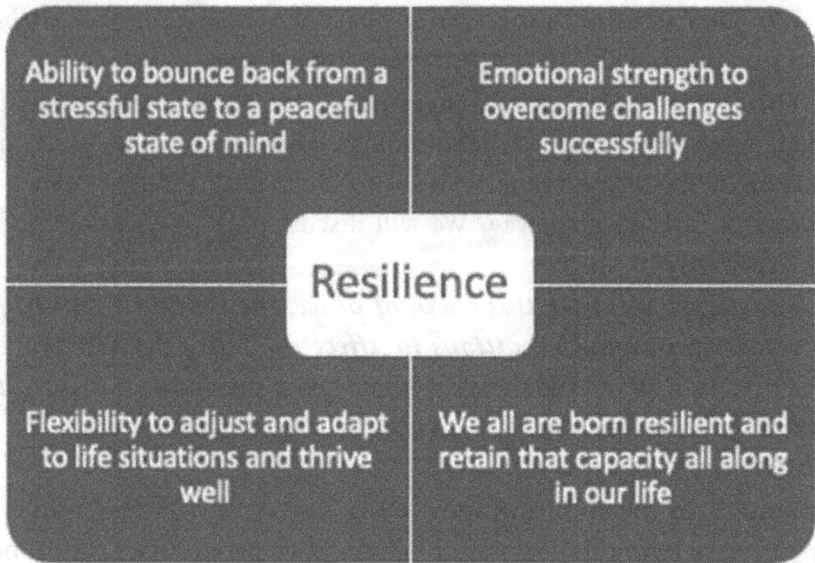

Figure 9

With the current situation with COVID, we all are going through an enormous amount of stress, whether it is health related, financial, or going crazy with home isolation. Some have lost their loved ones also. So, I understand it's not easy on you. ***But remember, you are your greatest asset. If you stay safe, healthy, and alive, you could always make the money back***. The top priority is to stay alive!

In summary, to bounce back from COVID-related stress, remember the following:

1. We all are born resilient. Resilience is your capacity to recover and heal from the stressful situations of life. It's your capacity to be flexible and adapt to life challenges.

2. Sometimes we get stressed. That's normal. But we don't have to stay stressed forever.

3. Being at peace and being joyful is your default setting. That makes it possible for you to recover from any kind of stress in life. You can overcome COVID stress also.

4. It is your innate potential to rebalance and restore peace, regardless of your circumstances.

5. As a resilient being, you are inherently designed to win. *The indomitable nature of human resilience has been proven time and again through the ages.* Tap into that inner power of yours.

The best time to further strengthen our resilience is during the time of crisis. Let's do that now. Let's face this together. Let's help each other. United we can defeat this pandemic.

Chapter 6:
How to Let Go of
Negativity

There is a lot of negativity right now in the world. Governments, big organizations, small businesses, employees, daily wage workers, health personnel, and other frontline workers...everyone is gripped by fear and anxiety. How do we come out of this negative state of thinking?

There are three things you need to understand:

- All negativity is created from within.
- The more you focus on it the more real it appears.
- Letting your thoughts flow washes away negativity.

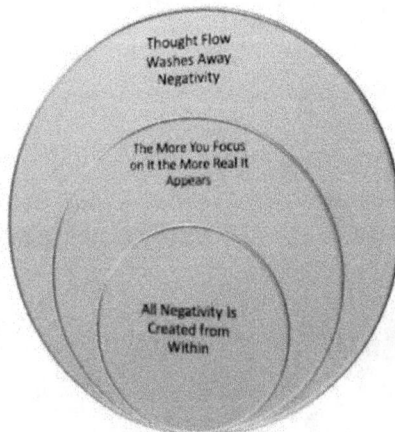

Thought Flow
Washes Away
Negativity

The More You Focus
on It the More Real It
Appears

All Negativity Is
Created from
Within

Figure 10

I.   *All negativity is created from within. It has little to do with what's going on outside you.* I know it is a little shocking to say that and probably I made you upset by this comment of mine. But *I can't help but tell you the truth. Truth is the only thing that liberates us.*

Let me give you an example. A couple of days ago, I was speaking with my gardener. I asked him how he was doing with this pandemic situation. His answer was, "I am doing all right. What can we do? We do our best and I believe everything will be all right." I was surprised by his answer. He is a daily wage worker, and it is probably not easy for him to take care of his family with a drop in income due to the economic impact of the pandemic. And yet, he has maintained a positive attitude. That's inspiring.

I also know people who are sitting at home and complaining constantly even though none of their family members or themselves are infected with coronavirus and they have enough money in reserves.

You see, *a lot has to do with our attitude toward the problem rather than the problem itself.* So, what I suggest is, if we develop a more positive attitude toward this crisis, it will help us do better. Of course, if you or one of your loved ones is in the Intensive Care Unit, that's a totally different situation. Also, if you have no money to buy food supplies, that's a difficult situation too. (We will address those two problems elsewhere in this book.) But if you are not in either of those categories, there is not much to complain about. We simply *adapt to the situation, lie low for a while, and move on.*

2.   This brings us to the question: How do we maintain a positive attitude when everything around us appears negative? The answer is simple: *Whatever you focus on appears real to you.* This can be explained using the TV and remote metaphor. If you watch a horror movie on TV, you feel horrified. If you watch a feel-good movie, you feel good. It's that simple! The remote to change the channels is in your hand. It's totally your choice. Our mind is like that.

If you choose to focus your mind on all the bad things that are happening out there, how many people died, how bad the situation is in

New York City, and how terrible this pandemic is, you will feel terrible. You will be pulled into a vortex of negativity and it may be very hard to come out of it. However, if you decide to focus on the fact that only four million out of the 7.7 billion population is infected and a vast majority is going to survive this pandemic, it makes you feel optimistic.

Here is an example. The other day, I was watching the documentary *Pandemic* on Netflix. I watched this almost six weeks into the pandemic. What I noticed was that I was more frightened by the events happening in the documentary than the COVID pandemic I had been dealing with the past few weeks. The narrators did a good job invoking the emotion of fear in me. I allowed that to happen by letting my mind be totally absorbed in it. There is an important lesson here. ***What you see on TV can be more frightening than what's actually happening in our day-to-day life. Differentiate those two.*** Our mind is powerful. It can magnify our emotions based on what we focus upon.

Choose where you want to focus your mind. The great thing is you have total control over where you want to focus your attention. Think about that!

I know, I know! You probably are going to say that controlling negative thoughts is not as easy as it sounds. But ***I am not telling you to control negative thoughts. I am simply saying that we should let go of them.*** Aren't both the same? No. There is a big difference.

When you try to control negative thoughts, you probably are trying to not think of something that's bothering you. But the more you try not to think of it the more it bothers you. For example, if you are telling yourself that you don't want to think of COVID and how deadly the disease is, you are already thinking about it. So, ***trying to get rid of the negative thoughts only potentiates them. Rather, you should simply ignore any negative thoughts that come to your mind.***

3. ***Thoughts flow in your mind like water flows in the river.*** As long as the river is free-flowing, the water is healthy to drink. The moment there is stagnation, the water gets dirty and unhealthy to drink. In the same way, if you let thoughts flow freely, your mind will remain healthy.

If you choose to hold on to negative thoughts, that causes stagnation in your mind and results in stress. When a negative thought comes to your mind, instead of latching onto it, ignore it so it will go away. These thoughts will have no choice but to leave if you decide not to give attention to them. Automatically, the next positive thought comes forth and washes away the negativity. The reason why so many people suffer with bad moods is because they brood over negative thoughts, whether they are COVID related or something else.

The solution is pretty simple—do not brood over negative thoughts. The more you practice this, the easier it becomes for you to let go of negativity. Also, purposefully focusing on something positive is an effective way to distract yourself away from negativity.

Despite knowing this, sometimes negative thoughts can be tenacious. During such situations, breathing exercises can be of great help. *Deep breathing slows down your thoughts. When your thoughts slow down, they become much more manageable.* Restlessness subsides and calmness prevails.

Do the following breathing exercise whenever you feel the need to calm down. I recommend at least 10 minutes in the morning and 10 minutes in the evening.

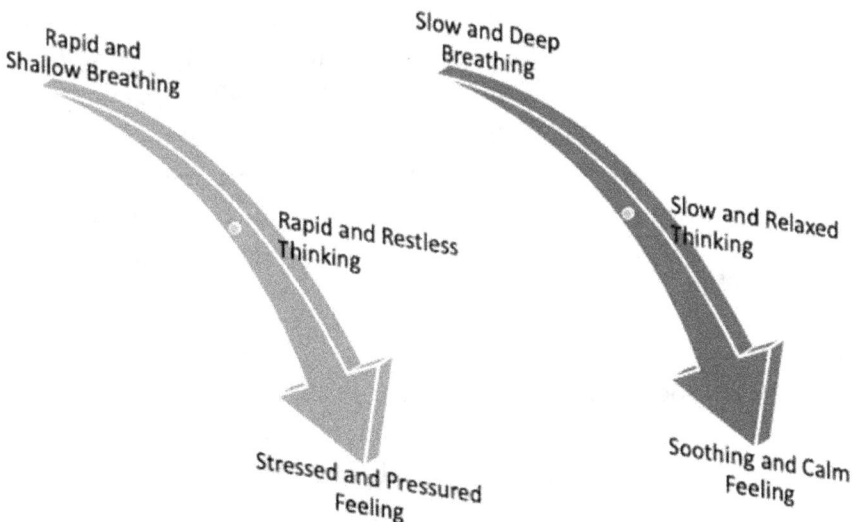

Figure 11

1. Lie down or sit back in an easy chair; completely relax both your mind and body. Just let go of everything—every thought, idea, limitation, pain, every past event, or future worry, every feeling, just about everything that could possibly arise in your mind—and just relax completely and ease into your body and mind.

2. Breathe deeply and release your breath slowly. Again, breathe deeply and release slowly. Do it a few times—possibly for the next few minutes. You feel your body and mind relaxing. Just ease into your breathing.

3. Let your breathing take a natural rhythm and follow it. Your breathing will slow down and will become very enjoyable and relaxing. Ease into it. Let it be. Let nothing bother you at this time. You are alone. You are free. You are enjoying yourself.

   a. Remind yourself that you have no limitations other than those you impose on yourself. As you breathe, notice that you can take only one breath at a time. Observe that one breath. Be in that moment; be in that breath completely.

   b. Then release the breath slowly, naturally. Be completely with it from the beginning to the end of the exhale. Observe it. Then let the next breath in. And continue the cycle. As you continue to do this, your breathing will slow down, your thoughts will slow down, and your awareness levels will rise.

   c. Whenever you lose the flow of observing your breathing, remind yourself that you can only take one breath at a time, that you can only either breathe in or breathe out; you can't do both at once. Then why jump forward and think about the next breath and the next moment? Stay with the breath and stay in the moment.

4. As you relax and ease into this state, you will feel all the restlessness in your body and mind completely dissolve. If you still feel a bit of restlessness, continue to ease into your breathing. Just let it be. If you want to, observe your breathing as it naturally happens.

5. Doing this exercise for five to 10 minutes is usually sufficient to completely relax you, but if you feel like you need to do it longer, that's fine too. But within the first five minutes, you may notice yourself falling into a sleeplike state in which you are deeply relaxed.

6. Rest there as long as you feel like before you return to your normal self. You will wake up feeling refreshed and rejuvenated. Now your mind is clear, and you can carry on with your daily activities.

Chapter 7:
Using Meditation to
Overcome COVID Stress

I had this experience in the midst of the corona pandemic.

There is nothing like meditation to help find solace during crisis. I just came out of deep meditation this morning. Felt so peaceful. Everything around me dissolved. Initially, I was restless. My thoughts were running astray in a thousand directions. But as I was determined to stay focused, my energy softened, and I entered a deep state of relaxation. After 20 minutes of effort (the phase of premeditation), all of a sudden, the restlessness disappeared. I slid into a trancelike state where nothing else existed. I was gone somewhere beautiful, peaceful, and joyful. That somewhere is within me, not outside me. Not an imagination. Not a visualization. It's a matter-of-fact thing. Then a thought came to me: "Why am I searching for peace and joy everywhere else? I should do more of this.

This world is such an illusion. It promises you to give happiness by instigating you to pursue material achievements only to realize that you fall flat in the process. Yes, you may even attain your goals, but it's a convoluted path laden with disappointments, disillusionments, and distress. After years of experience, I can wholeheartedly say that stress is the only guaranteed byproduct of your material pursuits, whether you succeed or not, whether you find happiness or not, whether you make money or not, whether you become famous or not. So, there is only one place to go to find true happiness, peace, and contentment.

That is within. That's where your true treasure is. So, let us go deeper in our inner journey to bring us closer to our true purpose in life, which is to find lasting peace, joy, and inner security in these times of great uncertainty.

COVID Meditation Technique:

To find solace quickly, I have simplified the meditation technique I regularly teach, to fit the needs of the people during this corona pandemic.

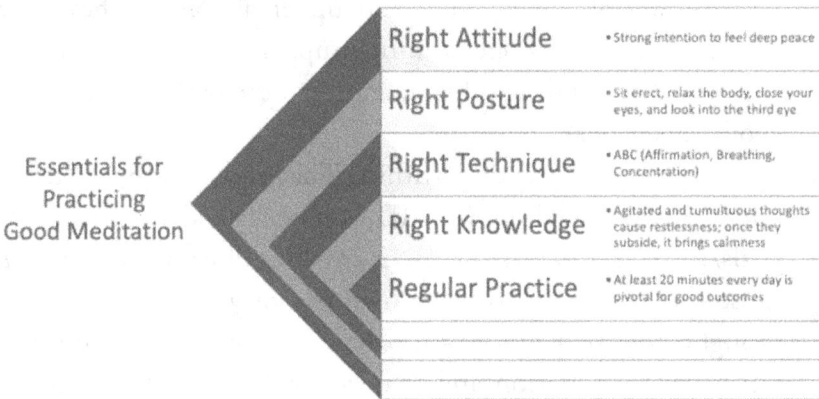

Essentials for Practicing Good Meditation		
	Right Attitude	• Strong intention to feel deep peace
	Right Posture	• Sit erect, relax the body, close your eyes, and look into the third eye
	Right Technique	• ABC (Affirmation, Breathing, Concentration)
	Right Knowledge	• Agitated and tumultuous thoughts cause restlessness; once they subside, it brings calmness
	Regular Practice	• At least 20 minutes every day is pivotal for good outcomes

Figure 12

A. Preparation:

1. Sit quietly in a place where no one can disturb you. If you have your own room, keep the door closed and let people know not to disturb you.
2. Be seated in a cross-legged posture on the floor if you can. If not, sit upright on a chair or any other firm surface.
3. The key to good meditation is to keep your spine erect, without letting it droop forward. That doesn't mean you have to tense your body. Keep your shoulders and back relaxed.

B. The Technique Proper:

1. **Sit upright with your spine erect and focus your gaze at the spiritual eye center,** the point between your two eyebrows.

Initially, it may be a little difficult because you are not used to it. With time, you will get used to it. Remember, no need to squint your eyes. Just slightly lift your gaze upward and forward. That will be sufficient.

2.   Once your attention is focused on the spiritual eye, **make sure your whole body is relaxed.** Instruct yourself to slowly and steadily relax each body part starting from: left foot-right foot, left leg-right leg, left thigh-right thigh, left buttock-right buttock, pelvis-lower abdomen, mid- and upper abdomen, chest, neck, and shoulders, left upper arm-right upper arm, left forearm-right forearm, left hand-right hand, and then the back. Feel the whole body totally relax.

3.   Now turn your attention within. That means, **stop thinking stuff** whether it is about COVID, your girlfriend/boyfriend, your goals/projects, financial issues, or anything else on your mind. All those thoughts need to be thrown out of your mind. Tell your thoughts that they can wait for the next 20-30 minutes until you finish your meditation and that you will attend to them later. Make sure you are still focused on your spiritual eye.

4.   Then **start feeling the peace within.** Remember that your true nature is peace. That is how you came into this world. You are born that way. As you grew into an adult, you somehow lost that peace, but it is waiting for you to come back. As your thoughts subside, the peace within swells up. Focus on that peace. Stay there.

5.   **Go deeper in your meditation.** Keep feeling the inner peace. If thoughts come to disturb you, gently push them away saying that you will return to them later, after the meditation. Every time you get disturbed, you keep bringing yourself back to the spiritual eye and the inner peace. **Chant the word "peace" and "visualize it" in your spiritual eye.** Keep focusing on it.

6.   At some point of time, **all thoughts cease to exist**. That is when you will feel a deep state of inner calmness, a sense of total security and total stillness. That's the experience you are looking for in your meditation. When you feel it, hold on to it as long as you can.

7. If you get disturbed by your thoughts, again **keep bringing yourself back** to this state of deep inner stillness and calmness. Sit there as long as you can, at least 10–15 minutes if not longer. The longer you sit in peace after practicing the technique, the greater its positive effects on you.

C. Post-meditation:

1. After the meditation session is concluded, slowly get up and move on with your daily activities. **Hold onto that calmness you experienced and carry it with you** wherever you go. Try to maintain calm throughout the day.

2. Do this technique **at least once in the morning and once in the evening** during this pandemic and you will see miracles happening in your life. You will carry a paradise of peace and joy within wherever you are and whatever your situation is.

D. Benefits:

1. **You will remain unruffled:** As you start doing this technique regularly, you will feel that even the pandemonium of crashing worlds cannot unsettle you. Your anxiety about coronavirus subsides. You will feel strong, courageous, and confident. Just make sure you practice this technique daily for the next 21 days without missing it even a single day.

2. **You will find prosperity:** When your mind is clear and your soul is at peace, automatically you will attract opportunities that help you succeed in life. However, when there is restlessness, you will create obstacles on your path inadvertently. Things that are supposed to work out start falling apart. But when you find deep calmness, even things that are falling apart will be mended. During these uncertain times, using this power of calmness is important for all of us to do well.

3. **You will feel secure:** During times of uncertainty, people feel very insecure about what's going to happen in their lives. That's only natural. However, by practicing this technique regularly, as you delve deeper into your inner self, you will feel a sense of certainty

and security that "all will be all right." You suddenly realize that you are complete and there is nothing to lose or nothing to be added to you for you to feel complete. That's the greatest feeling—a feeling that brings solace to your soul.

4. **You will sleep better:** People can't sleep properly because of anxiety or worry about some situation. Their restless thoughts constantly overstimulate their brain and make it hard for them to sleep. It is important to alleviate all this restlessness for us to sleep better. When your mind is calm and your soul at peace, you automatically rest your brain and sleep well.

Chapter 8:
Preventing Post-COVID Stress Disorder

Humanity is at a great risk for suffering from Post-COVID Stress Disorder (PCSD). Many people will likely end up having PCSD. We need to prepare ourselves now, to prevent it. But what is this PCSD? To understand that, you need to understand the difference between acute stress and chronic stress.

Acute stress is a normal physiological response we experience in the face of a threat. Your body secretes stress hormones like cortisol and adrenaline to help you face the threat or escape from it—the fight or flight response. Because of this, people feel anxiety and palpitations. They may also develop high blood pressure, chest pain, nausea, vomiting, dizziness, and many other symptoms. Some may even end up with a heart attack or stroke. In the medical community, we are already seeing this during this pandemic.

After the threat is over, the stress response should typically subside, and we should return to normal. However, we human beings do not let this stress go away. We often hold onto the traumatic events of the past or imagine a fearful future and perpetuate the stress. Let me give you an example. Many people who are not directly affected by the pandemic and who are not infected are very stressed sitting at home. This is true even after many weeks have passed since the beginning of the pandemic. Why is that? If none of your family members or you are infected and if you have enough financial reserves, why are you continuing to feel stressed?

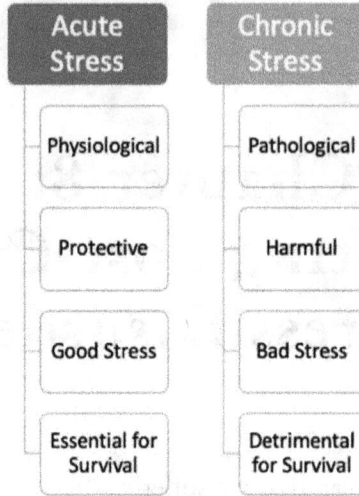

Acute Stress	Chronic Stress
Physiological	Pathological
Protective	Harmful
Good Stress	Bad Stress
Essential for Survival	Detrimental for Survival

Figure 13

It's because *our mind magnifies our suffering. We imagine the worst possible situations in our mind.* It's because we keep repeating in our mind how terrible this disease is and how horrible it is to be stuck in this situation, while sitting at home, far away from outbreak hotspots where the situation is really bad. Do you see my point? Even though there are some people who are directly affected, and they are totally justified to feel stressed out, *a vast majority of people who probably will never contract the virus are still suffering a lot mentally.* It's because, in their mind, "something horrible is happening or about to happen." This is greatly stirred up by constant exposure to bad news seen on TV. This is further made worse by *the weakness of human mind where it can't let go of bad news. We humans have the tendency to repeat negative thoughts in our mind forever like a CD that is stuck* and is playing the same song again and again. That's the reason for *chronic stress* in our lives.

Chronic stress results from a repetitive, dysfunctional thinking process in our mind. It has less to do with external circumstances and more to do with how we process the information we receive.

Let me give you an example that differentiates how we humans react compared to animals when it comes to stressful events.

Imagine a zebra is being hunted by a lion in Africa. Being hunted triggers an acute stress response in the zebra. Her heart races and pumps blood faster. Her lungs breathe rapidly. The energy stores are mobilized in her body so that she could run faster and escape from the lion. Hopefully, the zebra is lucky enough to escape. *After the zebra escapes, she comes to its normal state of being in 30-40 minutes. The acute stress response dissipates. She joins the herd, grazes, and moves along. This acute stress response is normal and physiological.* When we face a threat, it's normal to feel acutely stressed.

Now, imagine yourself in the same situation as the zebra. Let's say you went on an African safari trip. Despite the tour guide's warning, you strayed away from the group and encountered a lion, barely 20 feet away. You freeze. You start sweating, with your heart racing and feeling palpitations. You can't think straight. The lion smells your fear and takes a step forward, ready to lunge at you. You almost faint. Can't even move. You close your eyes, ready to be attacked by the lion any minute!

Then comes a banging sound from behind...the tour guide with his rifle scares away the lion. He finds you limp with no energy, your whole-body trembling. He takes you back to the tour bus. After an hour, finally, you stop sweating and shaking, coming back to your senses.

A bunch of tourists gather around, curious about your "safari experience." Though your body has calmed down, your mind has not. You are still thinking about the lion. You feel terrible about this whole "lion situation" you went through. You start cursing the lion. You start telling others how terrible this lion is and that all lions must be locked up and a safari tour is not a good idea as long as lions are freely roaming around. *To your dismayed audience, you go on narrating this terrible story of yours the whole day and you wonder why you continue to feel worse.*

Then you go back to your hotel room but that night you don't sleep well. You wake up from your dream in the middle of the night screaming that the lion is attacking you. Tossing and turning, unable to sleep, you call your family 10,000 miles away and tell them the terrible story, again. By morning, you feel so tired and irritable that you cancel your tour for that day. Though it was your lifelong dream to go on an African safari tour, you are not enjoying it anymore. You cancel the trip altogether to go back to your home country. Back home, you continue to tell this story whenever you get a chance. *Three months later, you still keep getting nightmares about the lion attacking you. Now, you've got Post-Traumatic Stress Disorder (PTSD).*

Do you see what the problem is here?

You continue to stress about an event that is no longer present. The lion has long forgotten you, but you haven't forgotten the lion. That's the problem.

That's the difference between the zebra who forgot the lion within an hour versus a human being who continued to brood over it for months, misusing his power of thinking. That's how we create chronic psychological stress in our lives...by repetitively thinking about stuff that happened in the past and sometimes, even worse, thinking about stuff that hasn't happened yet!

We use our thinking against ourselves and create suffering by obsessively repeating our thoughts. And the unfortunate thing is that we don't even realize that we are doing it to ourselves. It's an innocent mistake we make. It's because no one ever teaches us this stuff. But, once we realize that we are creating our own stress using our thinking against ourselves, we can stop doing that. Initially, it will be a little difficult because we are habituated to do that but in time we will succeed.

Extrapolating the above example to the coronavirus stress, when the World Health Organization (WHO) declared COVID as a pandemic, the whole world went into a state of terror. Everyone started panicking. That is acute stress response at a global scale. Mass hysteria followed. Now, what's happening is that our bodies and minds got used to the "threat" and the news of the pandemic. We all are settling down in home isolation and getting used to it.

Unfortunately, a vast majority of the population will continue to react badly to the COVID pandemic, even after it starts cooling down. We need to prevent that or else we will end up with a mental health pandemic in the form of Post-COVID Stress Disorder (PCSD). And we can only prevent that if we help people learn how to disconnect the link between acute stress and chronic stress. That link is "our thought." It is by stopping our minds from repeating negative thoughts that we remain sane and sound. We do that by practicing the teachings and techniques mentioned in the previous two chapters.

Chapter 9:
Recovering from the
Stress of Financial Loss

As of this writing, I am facing major financial problems like everyone else affected by the pandemic. My medical practice has suffered an almost 50% drop in revenue due to the pandemic. Also, there is not much financial reserve left in my portfolio. The retirement savings evaporated because of the stock market downturn. So, I am in the same boat as millions of others who are going through during this pandemic. So, I understand your pain. The financial hardship is palpable across all sections of the population—some less, some more—but everyone is affected in one way or another. So, what shall we do to come out of this? How can we stay calm during these trying circumstances? I will share with you what I am doing and how it is helping me do well.

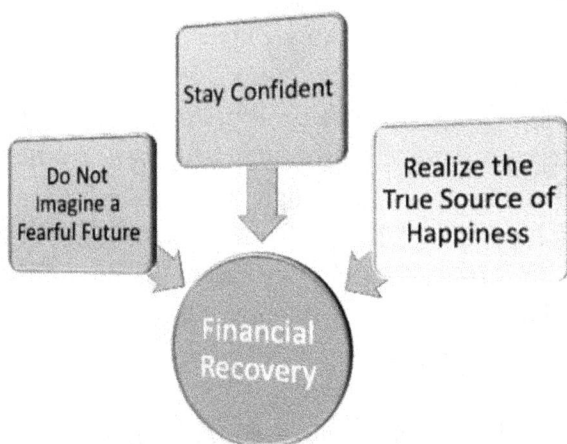

Figure 14

1. Stay Confident

I am 100% confident that things will turn around sooner or later. It's just a matter of time. We need to stay strong until this pandemic passes. If we need to borrow money, let us borrow; we can pay it off later. If banks do not want to give us money, I am sure there are enough good people in the world—whether your friend, family member, or neighbor—who will come to rescue. Let them know your situation and give them assurance that you will help them when they are in need. During these difficult times, most people will respond in kind. If your basic needs are taken care of over the next few months, the rest can be figured out later.

Yes, I know that many of you are worried about monthly payments of rent, mortgage, car payments, and other expenses. But what can you do if you don't have the money? The worst-case scenario is you are going to lose your car, home, and all the material possessions. I know it's not easy. But if you stay healthy and alive, you can make them all back.

When I came to the United States 15 years ago, I came with nothing and I quickly got into huge debt because I had to pay the tuition for higher studies. But with hard work, persistence, and diligence, I slowly paid off my debts and established a successful career. At that time, I was pursuing a teaching assistantship that paid me $940 per month and paid off my tuition for that semester. Everyone told me it was not possible and it was very hard to get, especially since the semester has already begun by the time I set the foot in the United States. Some of my friends listened to them but I didn't. I was deaf to their negative talk. I did what I had to. I was ingenuous, probably a little drastic, in creating my "first ever resume" so that people would take notice of it. Lo! There was unexpectedly a job opening, and because I was persistent and showed up at the biology department every other day, the secretary remembered my name and called me first even though there was a large pile of applications sitting in front of her! You can't imagine the joy I felt that day—my first victory in the United States. It gave me a lot of confidence that with hard work, persistence, and a little creativity, you can win against the odds in this land of opportunity.

During this time of COVID financial downturn, I am telling myself, "If I lose it all, I will make it back again. I am not afraid of hard work!" That kind of attitude helps us through these difficult times. What the heck! Let's not chicken out! Let's be strong. Let's be confident. All will be all right!

2. Do Not Imagine a Fearful Future

Everyone is affected including the largest economies of the world, major organizations, small businesses, employees, daily-wage workers, and more. So, do not think you are all alone in this. We are all in this together. We will all figure this out together.

We didn't expect such a bad financial downturn a few months ago, right? Then maybe there is going to be a giant financial upturn after this pandemic is over. Who knows? Then why imagine a fearful future? Stay optimistic. Hope for the best. Keep doing what you have to for your job or business.

More people are going to get into trouble because of the terrible future they are imagining than the financial downturn itself. Fear paralyzes people. It makes them do desperate things. An example of that is the German finance minister who committed suicide. It's quite unfortunate. But see that Germany is doing far better than many other countries. If he stayed alive, he would have seen that. So, do not lose your confidence. Do not lose your hope. Just stay put. The worst things that you are imagining may never come true. Perhaps you will not only make the money you lost but double the amount after this pandemic is over. Everything is possible if you just stay patient and wait for the right opportunity to bounce back financially.

3. Know the True Source of Your Happiness

Look, at the end of the day there is only one thing that is important— that's you. You are your own treasure. You accumulate all the other treasures, whether it is money, material possessions, stocks, or something else so that you can be happy, safe, and secure. *All those other treasures are there to support you, the real treasure. If you die, all those do not make any sense anymore. So, staying safe is more important than economy or money at this time.*

Man is in so much trouble right now because of his identification with money as the primary measure of success and happiness in life. To be honest, whether you are a CEO or a daily-wage worker, if your basic needs are fulfilled you should be all right. Everything else is secondary. There is enough food in this world to be distributed for all. The only thing that is preventing that from happening is greed and politics. I know there are people out there hoarding essential products so that they can sell them for a higher price later. They are artificially creating dearth of food. That's terrible. You see, *it is the greed and other terrible qualities in some people that is more detrimental to our survival than the pandemic itself.*

People need to realize that *"money is made for man, not man for money." When you came to this world, you came with nothing. When you leave this earth, you will leave with nothing.* Then why worry about what you accumulate in between? Unfortunately, we as a humanity have conditioned ourselves this way that we can't live without money. We are stuck in a greedy, overconsuming, and highly egoistic society that has identified its happiness with external things, and when they are lost, they feel that their life is worthless and that all they have is lost.

The truth is, your true happiness is within you. Maybe it's a good thing that we lost much of our money—that we suddenly realize that we can still be happy without it.

Let me give an example of that. Many years ago, when I was moving from Connecticut to California, we packed all the stuff at home and were ready for the move. We lived in a two-bedroom home at that time and we couldn't believe how much stuff we had accumulated in just a couple of years. Things kept coming out of nowhere when the movers came in. It took them double the time that was initially estimated. Finally, the house was totally emptied. It felt odd that night. We just slept on a thick blanket on the carpet, with a small pillow under our heads. Being tired, we had a very good night's sleep. But when we woke up the next morning, we realized we didn't have anything to eat. We quickly got some bagels and eggs along with orange juice from the store next to us. As we sat there eating breakfast, we came to the realization that even though all the stuff we had at home was gone, we still were happy and having a good day.

What happens if we lose all those goods? Will that make us unhappy? The immediate answer I got from within was, *No! Not at all.* In fact, I felt like they were encumbrances. To say it in another way, *It's too much crap!* We accumulate it for some unknown reason. The point is, our happiness is not dependent on that "crap." It lies within us. It depends on our attitude. It depends on how we treat each other as human beings. It depends on how kind we are toward others. When we realize that, automatically our attachment to material possessions falls away. You may still buy things and accumulate stuff, but you won't be dependent on them for your happiness.

When we are like that, we will be truly happy. As of today, I am seriously thinking to adopt this new lifestyle—simple living, getting rid of everything I don't need, and downsizing to a small place. Let's see if I can make it happen ☺

Chapter 10:
Staying Sane During
Home Isolation

With total lockdown, so many people are going crazy during this pandemic. People are not used to sitting at home and doing nothing. Humans are social beings, and all of a sudden their social interactions are truncated to the minimum. Instead of becoming frustrated with the situation, there are things to do that can help you.

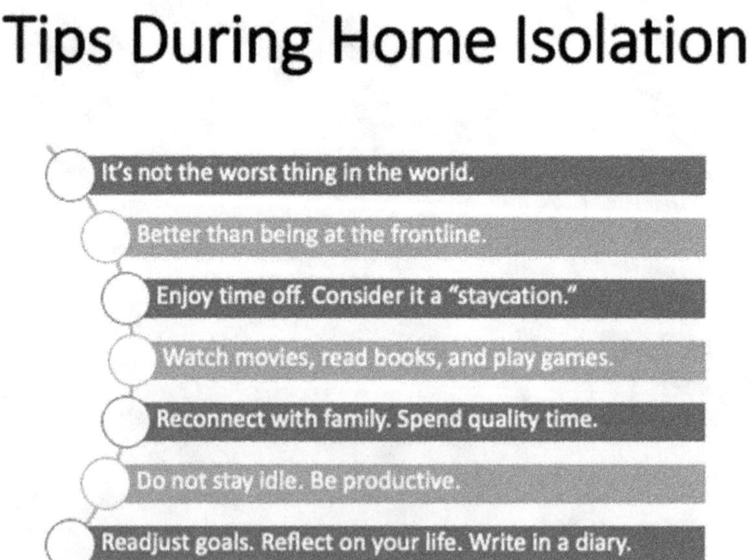

Tips During Home Isolation

It's not the worst thing in the world.

Better than being at the frontline.

Enjoy time off. Consider it a "staycation."

Watch movies, read books, and play games.

Reconnect with family. Spend quality time.

Do not stay idle. Be productive.

Readjust goals. Reflect on your life. Write in a diary.

Figure 15

I. Remember, being stuck at home is better than being at the frontline.

1. It is **not the worst thing in the world** to be isolated at home. Let's appreciate the doctors, nurses, and others risking their lives for us. Imagine what kind of difficulties our frontline workers are going through because of COVID.

2. They are **at a great risk of exposing themselves to sick patients**, especially those without appropriate Personal Protective Equipment (PPE). Yet, they have to heroically go save others' lives, risking their own.

3. Even more worrisome for them is that when they go home, they are **not sure if they are carrying the virus and may be infecting their families.** There is no sure way to know it. Also, we in the health care profession see many patients, and because most of the COVID patients are asymptomatic, we may have been even exposed to the virus without ever knowing about it.

4. So, when you think about all that, you suddenly realize that getting stuck at home and **being safe is far better than going out** and getting exposed to the virus. For the next many weeks to months, maintain this perspective. It will help you.

II. Enjoy your time off.

1. **I know it's difficult to be stuck at home.** But what can you do? Everything is closed. Don't we always complain that we don't have enough time for important things in our personal lives because we are so busy at work?

2. Consider this to be the long **two-month vacation** that you always wanted. Consider this a staycation!

3. Fortunately, we have so many options for **home entertainment** these days. With a little bit of thinking and planning, you can turn the home isolation into an enjoyable HOME VACATION.

4. Maybe, this is the time to **watch all your favorite movies** and shows.

5. **Reconnect with your family** and friends that you have long forgotten.

6. How about **reading some books?** My favorite is fiction. I haven't read any suspense thrillers in a long time. I am going to do that now. Do whatever works for you. Have fun.

7. Play **videogames** if that's your thing.

I have one warning, though. Don't overdo watching movies and playing videogames. Too much screen time will strain your eyes and you may develop dry eyes. You don't want that. Also, those who play videogames nonstop may develop carpal tunnel syndrome (CTS) and repetitive strain injury (RSI). Do everything in moderation and you will remain healthy.

III. Do not stay idle. Be productive. That's my strong recommendation.

An idle man's brain is the devil's workshop. Instead of going crazy, use this opportunity to get things done that you have been postponing. If you are someone worried that you are losing productive time because of the pandemic, here are five ways to stay productive during the COVID pandemic:

1. **Do some goal setting,** especially if you missed setting your New Year's resolutions.
   a. Goals have the power to drive you forward and help you accomplish what you need to in life.
   b. Reflect upon what you have done so far this year and what else needs to be done.
   c. Considering the unexpected changes due to the pandemic, see if you need to readjust your targets.
   d. ADAPT! ADAPT! ADAPT! That's the key to our survival.

2. **Rebuild your relationships.** We are so busy in the modern world that we do not give enough time to our loved ones.
   a. This is a perfect time to bond with your spouse, children, parents, or other family members.
   b. One of the major reasons for relationship fallouts is lack of proper understanding between people.
   c. And this happens because we don't truly listen to others. We often cite lack of time as an excuse. Well, it's no longer an excuse.

d. We have all the time in the world now. Use this time to practice listening and truly understanding your family members. This will heal your relationships. It will greatly enrich your life.

3. **If you enjoy reading spiritual or self-help books, go for it.**
   a. *There is no better time than a crisis to learn something new and rebuild yourself.*
   b. *Use this crisis to get stronger, not weaker.* In fact, reading books is one of the best things you can do during home isolation. It is a sure way to develop a good personality and enlighten ourselves with new knowledge.
   c. Books have the capability to open our minds to new ideas and expand our perspective.

4. **How about getting your home back in order?**
   a. You could unclutter your closet, clear up your desk, and organize your files. So much can be done if you stay calm and use your time wisely.
   b. Often, many people's closets are full of stuff they never use. How about sorting through all your clothes and donating the ones you don't use.
   c. Gardening is another way to go. Many people derive great pleasure when they work in nature and take care of plants. I decided to plant some greenery in our backyard. I am looking forward to it.

5. **Exercise and reclaim your physical health.**
   a. I know fitness clubs and yoga studios are closed but you could still do yoga or some kind of workout at home. There are so many YouTube videos to help with selecting an exercise regimen that fits you.
   b. How many of us complain that we don't get enough time to exercise? Most of us do not even spend 20 minutes a day on exercise. Well, now you have enough time. But I still see that so many people are not exercising.

    c. Do you see now that actually it is your habits that prevent you from exercising than time itself? This is the time then to build a strong habit of exercising daily.

    d. How about safe, outdoor activity that provides ample fresh air and sunshine? Consider exercising in the backyard.

    e. Playing ball with the kids, jogging, bike riding, and lots of walks are other options to consider, if you are able to maintain a safe distance and wear masks in densely populated areas. Perhaps go out in the early morning and in the evening when there are fewer people. All of this is great for stress-relief.

V. **Maintain Balance:** Some people are worried about their lives being totally out of balance during the pandemic. That is a valid concern. It is essential that we maintain some balance in our lives while staying in home isolation. Here is how to find good work–life balance during COVID:

    I. **Balance is a matter of perspective.**

        a. You need to redefine what balance means for you during this crisis.

        b. If you are working from home, it may be hard to draw a sharp line between work and home activities. Probably you got to do both at the same time.

        c. With schools closed, you may even have to babysit. You need to exercise at home.

        d. For all of this, a little planning will be helpful.

    2. **Divide tasks between yourself and your family members.**

        a. Delegate when you have to, but multitasking will be needed here.

        b. A calm mind can multitask easily. But a restless mind can't even do one task properly because a restless mind is distracted and error-prone.

        c. So, it is time to calm your mind. A calm mind is an efficient mind. Spend at least 10 minutes in the morning and 10 minutes in the evening relaxing your mind. If possible, make it 30 minutes in the morning and 30 minutes in the evening.

    d. Relaxation exercises are a powerful way to calm your mind. They ease tension in your body and make you feel more energetic.

3. **Ensure your gym time, work time, and family time are sharply demarcated.**
   a. Schedule the activities on your calendar. Have the discipline to follow through.
   b. Some amount of overlap is unavoidable because we are stuck in home isolation but do your best to demarcate them.
   c. Be flexible with your time slots. Shuffle them around and make it work for you.
   d. Have two or three major tasks you need to accomplish each day and make sure you do them first thing in the morning, if possible.
   e. Explain to your family and kids that this is how your schedule looks today and you expect some privacy to finish those.
   f. Reciprocate the same courtesy to other working members at home. Give them time to finish their chores too.

4. **Don't work nonstop, just because you are working from home.**
   a. Take a break when needed or else you will get fatigued. Sitting in front of the computer for a long time is not good for your spinal health.
   b. Most people stuck to their desks develop early degenerative changes in their neck and back, leading to chronic neck/back pain. People also get headaches because of constant work.
   c. It is easy to lose track of time and work yourself to death when working from home. Many of my friends are reporting that it is much harder to work from home because you really don't know how to stop working.
   d. When we go to the office, we socialize, we get up for coffee or lunch. However, all those natural breaks in office time are nonexistent at home, unless you schedule them purposefully.
   e. So, take a scheduled break at least once every 30 minutes for five minutes or once every hour for 10 minutes.

5. **It's perfect time to resurrect your lost cooking skills** and have a healthy home-cooked meal, as most restaurants are closed. I am already seeing many families doing that. Maybe we can continue this even after the pandemic is over.

See, the point is that a lot of things can be done to enjoy our time and be productive during home lockdown. We as human beings have the ability to adapt and adjust to life challenges. We can redefine our perspectives. We can change. That's our greatest strength. Let's use it to our advantage.

Chapter 11:
Preventing Relationship Breakdowns

Because of the corona crisis and home isolation, people are stuck at home. Staying home together for a long time is new for many couples. Usually, we wake up, go to work, come home in the evening, spend a little time together, and then we go to sleep. That has changed with home isolation. There is a drastic increase in personal contact between couples. This is good in some ways, but it can lead to increased conflict also. Maybe for the first time, you are seeing certain traits in your spouse that you were totally unaware of and you are shocked. But wait! Do not judge yet. Do not let those imperfections break your relationships. No one is perfect. Like you are seeing imperfections in others, probably they are seeing them in you too. Take time. Step back. Do not make any rash decisions now. Let this pandemic pass. Then you could reflect upon your relationship dynamics more peacefully and make wise decisions.

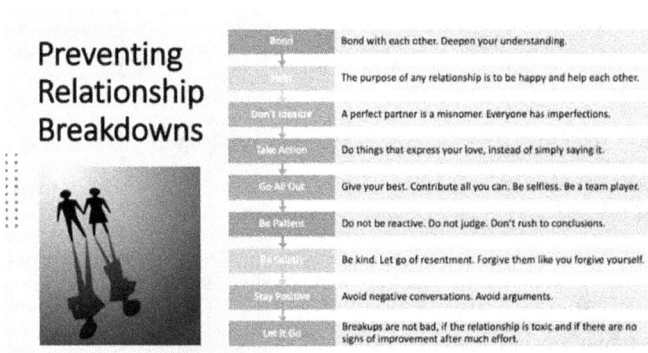

Preventing Relationship Breakdowns

Bond	Bond with each other. Deepen your understanding.
	The purpose of any relationship is to be happy and help each other.
Don't Idealize	A perfect partner is a misnomer. Everyone has imperfections.
Take Action	Do things that express your love, instead of simply saying it.
Go All Out	Give your best. Contribute all you can. Be selfless. Be a team player.
Be Patient	Do not be reactive. Do not judge. Don't rush to conclusions.
Be Saintly	Be kind. Let go of resentment. Forgive them like you forgive yourself.
Stay Positive	Avoid negative conversations. Avoid arguments.
Let It Go	Breakups are not bad, if the relationship is toxic and if there are no signs of improvement after much effort.

Figure 16

Guidance for Couples During the Corona Pandemic

1. Corona has provided us with an opportunity like never before to get to know our loved ones better. Normally, we are so busy with work and business obligations and have little time for each other.
2. What normally takes years to get to know each other now probably can be known in days to weeks during home isolation.
3. If you are not married and are in a live-in relationship, this is the perfect time to get to know the positives and negatives about your partner.
4. If you are already married, this is the time to deepen your understanding between each other.
5. But remember, if you are expecting the other person to be perfect all the time, it's not going to happen. Do not idealize your relationships.
6. A perfect partner is a misnomer. Initially, you may feel that person is perfect, but with time you will notice things that are less than perfect.
7. Instead of looking for perfection in your partner, look for signs of love and affection. As long as that is there, you could still work on improving yourselves.

Why Breakups Are Not Always Bad

1. What we thought to be a perfect relationship at one point of time may become the most toxic relationship as months and years pass by. This is not uncommon. It may be one person's fault, or it may be because of both people involved in the relationship. It could be because of the influence of in-laws, friends, etc.
2. See if you could resolve the difficult situations you are facing. First, see if you have given the best you can and if there is anything you can do to change yourself. Next, see if there is willingness from the other person to change and improve themselves in a way that is beneficial to the relationship.
3. Remember, you can't clap with one hand. Both people must be ready to contribute and improve the relationship. If you see the other person is not ready to be a *team player*, despite your repeated requests, that's a red flag.

4. If the relationship is failing despite repeated attempts to make it work, maybe it's time to move on. The time frame for making a relationship work has to be determined by your own personal situation. But one thing is true. Be patient. Do not jump to quick conclusions. Do not make hasty decisions. I have seen relationships heal with time. Time is the greatest healer—if you can really give yourselves that time.

5. Sometimes, breaking up is better if you are constantly living in a toxic environment that's harmful for you and the others involved. If it comes to that, move on peacefully. Two people may still remain friends even though they can't be spouses. And that is all right. The purpose of a relationship is to be happy and to learn from each other. If neither of them is possible, maybe it is better to move on.

Five Rules to Maintain Stable Relationships During the Pandemic

1. **Avoid negative conversations.** This pandemic has brought a lot of stress into our lives. Regardless of the reason, when we are stressed, we tend to gravitate toward negativity. We easily get into arguments. If you find yourself in such situations, silently excuse yourself from there. Let them know you will come back a little later.

2. **Be kind to others.** Give them the benefit of doubt even when you think they are wrong. In close relationships, it is okay to take a step back and let the other person have their way, as long as it is not harming you. We often think that by being tough and assertive we can change others. It actually works the other way around. Your kindness will transform them faster than your meanness.

3. **Show love in action.** We may express our love toward others in words, but words lose their power if they are not supported by our actions. Sometimes, when we are struggling in our relationships, our words may not convince others of our love toward them, but our actions will. Look for opportunities to express your love through your deeds.

4. **Let go of resentment.** For any reason if you have a strained relationship at home, at least for the time being, let go of all anger and resentment. Remember, resentment is like a hot charcoal. The longer you hold it, the greater your pain will be. For the next few months, treat each other normally. Maybe things will turn around by the time this pandemic is over.

5. **Forgive others as you would forgive yourself.** We find it quite easy to forgive ourselves even when we make big mistakes. Yet, we don't forgive others so easily. We see others' faults through a magnifying glass, and we minimize our own. When you turn that around and start being more forgiving toward people, you will develop a saintly personality.

Chapter 12:
How to Calm Your Child During a Crisis

COVID-19 has not only affected adults but has also affected our children. Schools are shut down. Parks, museums, and playgrounds are closed, leaving our children with nowhere to go. The home isolation by itself is hard on us, and if you have to work from home and still take care of your child, it's even more challenging. Children need constant attention. They are energetic and want to expend it by playing games or going out and spending time with their friends. As it's not possible now, they can get impatient at home. Also, they may be anxious about why everything is closed and why they can't go anywhere. It's easy to get irritated by their questions, especially when you are already under a lot stress because of the pandemic. Also, you may be concerned about your child's health during this crisis. I have a five-year-old daughter at home. So, I understand your struggles.

Here are some pointers for you as a parent to alleviate your child's anxiety during COVID.

1. First, know that COVID is predominantly seen in adults. Children are minimally affected and may have only mild symptoms. Deaths in children are extremely rare. (This may change with time as we know more about this disease). Ask your children to take necessary precautions as you do. Lead them by example.

2. If your child gets anxious, explain to them in simple terms what's going on with COVID. Explain that a majority of people,

over 98.6%, recover (per New York City data as of May 1) https://www.
worldometers.info/coronavirus/coronavirus-death-rate/.   Reassure
them that everything will be all right.

3. Control your own anxiety. Do whatever is needed to help yourself
    calm down. If you can't calm yourself, how can you calm your child?
    Children follow what you do, not so much what you say.
4. Distract your children and yourself from the negativity seen on TV
    and social media. Watch feel-good movies together. Spend family
    time. Read an inspirational story.
5. Make sure you as well as your children sleep well. That boosts your
    immunity and keeps the infection at bay.

Personally, the home isolation situation and the corona crisis worked very
well for me, when it came to bonding deeply with my daughter. Instead of
getting frustrated about the situation, we used it to our advantage. Every day
we would wake up, quickly have breakfast, and get ready for the day. If I have
to make any phone calls or be in a virtual conference, I would tell her not to
disturb me and I would give her some activities to do before I got on the call.

I have found that if we tell children ahead of time what to expect,
they are pretty good at understanding and following our instructions.
After a couple of hours of work from home, I take my daughter for a
bike ride or a walk. Then we have lunch and again get back to work
while she does some learning activities. Later in the afternoon, we watch
a movie or something else she likes on TV. Or we play a videogame
together. She loves Angry Birds! So, it has been a great experience for me.
I have learned a lot about my daughter these past two months. Normally,
I wouldn't get so much free time with her.

So, the point is, even when things are going south, we can make it work
for us by shifting our perspective and using our time and resources to the
best of our abilities. Don't think I am able to do all this because I am getting
a stable income. That's not true. I have lost more than 50% of income and
I have other problems in life too. But I resolved to not be drowned by the negativity around us and I will continue to do my best through this pandemic.

Initially, when my daughter asked what's going on, I explained to her
about the coronavirus in simple terms. She understood enough to know

that we should not go to public places and if we do, we should not touch anything unnecessarily, we should wear a mask, and we should wash our hands. For the first couple of trips, it was a struggle. She didn't want to wash her hands when we came home, and she touched everything. But with a little bit of explaining she got the point.

Handling a toddler is one thing but handling a teenager is a completely different thing. Having a teenager at home can be challenging even during normal times. During these extremely stressful times, it can be even more challenging. Here is what you can do.

Handling Teenagers During Crisis

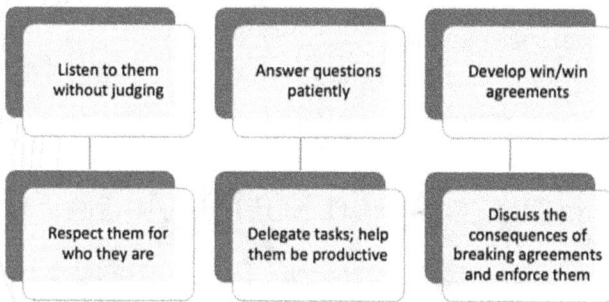

Listen to them without judging	Answer questions patiently	Develop win/win agreements
Respect them for who they are	Delegate tasks; help them be productive	Discuss the consequences of breaking agreements and enforce them

Figure 17

1. Most teenagers listen to you if you respect their perspective, without dismissing them altogether. Respect them for who they are and what they have to say about the situation.
2. I know it is difficult, but I still ask you to be patient with your teens. It helps both of you. Answer any questions they have, patiently.
3. If you have to use your parental authority to prevent them from going out into crowds, it's time to do so. But do so gently.
4. Develop win/win agreements with your teenagers. Discuss the consequences of breaking the agreement and enforce the agreement.
5. Delegate some tasks to them during this busy time. That will distract them from their phones and help be productive.

When I was growing up, there was not much on TV. There was no social media. Whatever happened at school and home is all I knew. But these days, the teenagers are being exposed to so much negativity. There is a constant barrage of bad news on TV. The worse the news, the more sensational it is. The news channels ramp up their sensationalism and we get pulled into the negativity, sitting at home watching TV intently.

Teenagers are affected even more because their minds are vulnerable, and they tend to believe all that they see. Also, there is so much negativity on social media. Teenagers these days spend a ton of time on Instagram, Facebook, and other platforms. Any bad event happening even tens of thousands of miles away immediately reaches them and volatile comments spread like a wildfire on social media. As a result, there is a tremendous amount of anxiety, worry, fear, anger, hatred, and other negative emotions being absorbed from social media.

Here are some ways on how to protect yourselves and your children from social media stress:

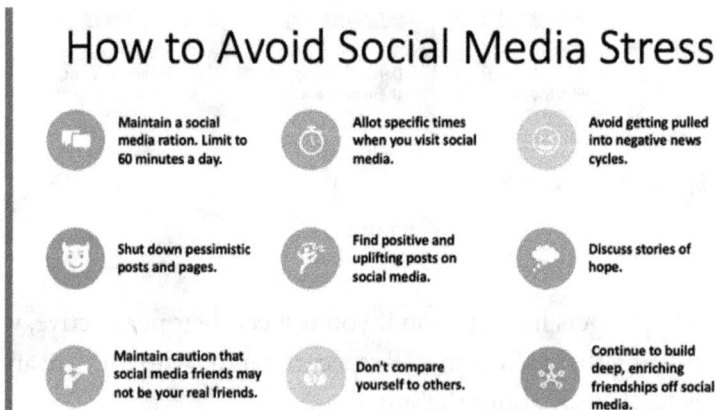

How to Avoid Social Media Stress

Maintain a social media ration. Limit to 60 minutes a day.

Allot specific times when you visit social media.

Avoid getting pulled into negative news cycles.

Shut down pessimistic posts and pages.

Find positive and uplifting posts on social media.

Discuss stories of hope.

Maintain caution that social media friends may not be your real friends.

Don't compare yourself to others.

Continue to build deep, enriching friendships off social media.

Figure 18

1. **Maintain social media ration.** Not more than 30 minutes in the morning and 30 minutes in the evening.
2. **Allot specific times when you will visit social media.** Let your social media friends know about this new initiative you have taken. Stick to it.

3. **Avoid being pulled into negative news cycles.** Shut yourself away from those pages if you can.

4. **Find positive and uplifting posts on social media** and be an advocate for them.

5. **Maintain caution** that social media friends may not be your real friends.

6. **Don't compare yourself to others.** Know that just because someone posted a happy picture on Facebook, it doesn't really mean they are happy.

7. **Continue to build deep, enriching friendships off social media** and eventually your dependence on social media lessens.

Chapter 13:
Overcoming Grief and Finding Solace

(This is a topic that I do not tread on usually but I decided to do so now because there are so many people affected by the coronavirus pandemic and have lost their loved ones. I hope to bring some solace to you with my commentary below on life and death. As a physician, I typically stay away from topics that I cannot provide scientific evidence. But when it comes to death, we will never have enough scientific evidence. We've got to base our discussions on our personal experiences and beliefs.)

Of all the emotions, grief is the one I have greatest respect for. Grief is the most difficult one to overcome because we can't see our loved ones who crossed the threshold over to the great beyond. ***Grief is mixed with love, for without love there is no grief***. It's hard to get over it. I know this by personal experience. There are times when no one will be able to console you, despite their best efforts. Then how do you overcome grief? How do you get back to normal? How do you move on with your life while the memories of your loved ones are still fresh in your mind? Sometimes these memories can be there with you not just for weeks or months, but for years. So, ***how do we hold on to the good memories while letting go of the painful ones, especially when both are tightly amalgamated?*** How do you let go of the emotional anguish? These are difficult questions. Sometimes no matter what others say, our hearts are not ready to heal. We need more time to let go. Time is the greatest healer in such situations.

Life and death are two sides of the same coin. When we are alive, we don't know what it is to be dead; when we are dead, we are not alive anymore. No wonder there is so much mystery about death. But all those who live must die at some point. That's inevitable. We can all agree on that. So, what matters is how well we live while we are alive. Anything beyond, we just don't know. When we don't know what is beyond, we are left to speculate. But it is not best to speculate on such great mysteries. *Rather, if we understand life, it makes it easier to understand death.*

If we look at human life, we come to this earth with nothing and we leave the earth with nothing. Who are we when we are born? Are we just flesh and bones? If we are just flesh and bones, how were we created? Who created us? Of course, the easy answer is when the sperm and ova reproduce, it leads to life. The single cell of life replicates itself into an embryo, then into a fetus, and then continues to develop into a little baby—that's you— and comes into this world as a newborn. Then you continue to grow into a toddler, a child, an adolescent, and finally into an adult. Then you continue with your life into middle age and old age until finally you die. That's the life and death cycle.

Where does life come from and where does it go after death? If life is something we can create, then by now we would have created it. You may say that we are creating life using "test-tube babies" or "*in vitro* fertilization," but still we are using the preformed egg and sperm from donors to **spring** life out of them. But what is it in our cells that breathes life into them? If it is just RNA and DNA that create life, our scientists have already figured out how to synthesize these individual components, yet they could not create cells with its complex structures, mitochondria, Golgi apparatus, lysosomes, and more. What about the myriad of cells that differentiate exactly into bones, muscles, brain, heart, eyes, and many more highly specialized cells that exactly serve a specific function? Who is creating all that? Not us, right? It's not like you were telling your body to develop into these components. All these processes are happening within and we are not even aware of it. So, can we claim ourselves to be the creators? Then what creates us? *Is there an intelligence that secretly operates behind the scenes and directs our cellular machinery to work harmoniously? What is that intelligence? I call it life. Life happens to us.*

Life is that intelligent force that creates us, sustains us, and ultimately withdraws from us when the time is ripe. No one knows exactly for sure when their time has come to leave this body. But as we grow from little babies into adults, we develop our own ideas about this world based on our interactions with this world. We develop emotions and attachments to the people in our life. They become part of us. We soon come to believe that we can't live without them, whether it is your son, daughter, mother, father, spouse, or friend. But isn't it true that once we lived without them, without having any attachment to them? This is especially true when it comes to friendships and spousal relationships. Then where is this attachment coming from? Is it because of the familiarity with the person? Is it because of the good things they have done for us? My answer is yes! We only grieve for people whom we love. And we love those people who are good to us, who cared for us, and who sacrificed themselves for us. *So, we can agree that grief arises from attachment to the person we love.*

Tips for Overcoming Grief and Finding Solace – I

Grief is admixed with love, for without love there is no grief.

Grief is directly proportional to the degree of attachment to our loved ones.

The initial grief is because we feel sad that the person's life has come to an end.

Everyone is different and everyone heals at their own pace.

Be kind to yourself. It is important during these times to not to be hard on yourself.

Hold on to the good memories and let go of the painful ones.

Life and death are two sides of the same coin.

We come to this earth with nothing and we leave with nothing.

Life is that intelligent force that creates us, sustains us, and ultimately withdraws from us when the time is ripe.

Figure 19

Why do we grieve for our loved ones? Is it because of our loss or their loss? When we lose our loved ones there is sorrow because we miss them. We would love to spend more time with them. We remember all the beautiful moments with them. We wish they were still there with us. So, are

Tips for Overcoming Grief and Finding Solace – II

Understand that we are not mere bodies but actually more than that.

If we can calm our minds and stop the dance of the restless thoughts, we will find peace, at least momentarily.

Meditation is one of the greatest healers when it comes to grief.

Read scriptures and spiritual books. They are of great value.

Do not blame people who trying to help you.

If there is someone who can truly understand what you are going through, it will ease your pain significantly.

We can't bring back our loved ones who have passed to the great beyond. And our own suffering will not bring happiness to them either.

Exercise regularly or else your body will decondition.

Take care of yourself, improve your emotional well-being, and carry on with your daily activities.

Figure 20

we grieving the lack of their presence and our dependence on them for us to be happy, to be loved, and to feel complete? If so, are we grieving for them or for ourselves? When I look deeper, I find both to be true.

The initial grief is because we feel sad that the person's life has to come to an end. This is especially true when our loved ones leave us abruptly, like a premature death due to an accident, an illness, or suicide. The grief is typically less when our loved ones had a good long life and the time is ripe for them to leave. Also, our grief is directly proportional to the degree of attachment to our loved ones.

With time, the grief we feel slowly lessens and sometimes it may take years before it gets totally resolved. What do we do until then? Are there ways to ease the grief?

If we understand that we are not mere bodies but actually more than that, it helps a lot to ease our grief. If we understand that we are souls who have come on to this earth for a purpose and that we leave this earth when that purpose is fulfilled, it brings us some solace. Otherwise, sometimes it doesn't make sense why a young boy who has not seen much life dies abruptly of disease or accident. What wrong has he done? Probably nothing. Then why does it happen? No one knows. Things happen in life for a variety of reasons.

Sometimes there is nothing we can do but live with our loss and wait for the grief to ease. Often, during those times, our emotions are out of our control. Our thoughts fly in a thousand directions. Our memories intrude into everything we do. *During these times, if we can calm our minds and stop the dance of the restless thoughts, we will find peace, at least momentarily.* That momentary peace can be slowly expanded into a much deeper state for longer periods of time. *When we are able to rise above the gravity of our emotion and when we are able to detach ourselves from the situation at least for a little while each day, it brings great relief.*

Meditation is one of the greatest healers when it comes to grief. Meditation aids you in accessing the PEACE behind your thoughts. It helps dissolve the sorrow by softening the painful memories and retaining the fond ones. It gives you insights into the nature of your soul. It shows things in a new light. As new understanding dawns upon you, it eases your suffering.

Reading scriptures and spiritual books is also helpful during these times. They can be your best friends. You can be totally lost in those books for a while and forget the loss of your loved ones at least during that time.

During this agonizing time, your friends and family will try to console you. They will tell you to forget the past and move on. But often, it's hard to move on. Sometimes what they say may make you feel hurt, though that's not their intention. Do not blame them. They are just trying to help you.

On one side, you may want to move on, and on the other side, you feel pulled back by your memories. It's all right. Take your time. *Everyone is different and everyone heals at their own pace. What is important during these times is not to be hard on yourself.* Do not blame yourself. Embrace new friendships. Spend more time with people who understand you.

Understanding is one of the greatest healers during these times. If there is someone who can truly understand what you are going through, it will ease your pain significantly. Keep moving forward with life.

Exercise regularly or else your body will decondition. Severe emotional pain can disrupt your bodily processes and can lead to diseases that you never thought were possible. For example, people with severe emotional pain can develop stress cardiomyopathy, where your heart becomes dilated and weak. You develop symptoms of congestive heart failure.

This happened to my uncle when he lost his mother. He eventually came out of it as his grief resolved.

So, the point is, we need to protect ourselves, improve our emotional well-being, and carry on with our daily activities during these difficult times to the best of our ability, no matter how deep our loss is. We can't bring back our loved ones who have passed to the great beyond. And our own suffering will not bring happiness to them either. So, it is important that we do everything to ease our suffering. Please do so. Be kind to yourself.

Chapter 14:
Five Recommendations on How to Safely Reopen the Economy

The coronavirus pandemic pushed the whole world into a state of chaos. The United States, the world's largest economy, has come to a standstill. People are struggling financially. If we don't reopen the economy, more people are going to die of starvation than the virus itself. Civil war may break out. Already there are large protests across the country. So, what's the solution? How soon should we reopen the economy and what's the best way to do it? Here is how:

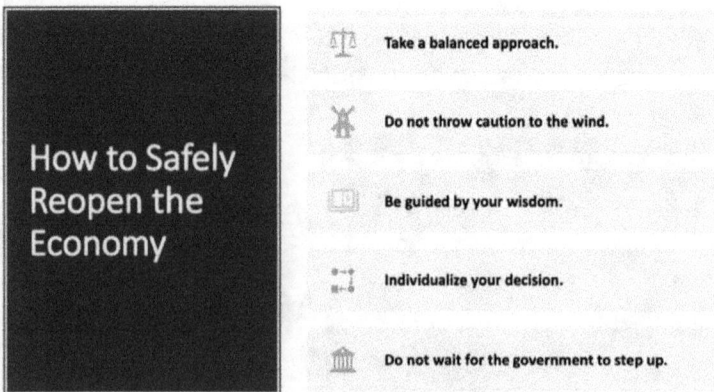

How to Safely Reopen the Economy

Copyright: Dr. Kevin Dimkpala

- Take a balanced approach.
- Do not throw caution to the wind.
- Be guided by your wisdom.
- Individualize your decision.
- Do not wait for the government to step up.

Figure 21

1. **We Need to Take a Balanced Approach.**
    a. We should look at this not only from a medical perspective but also from an economic perspective. We must understand the woes of the common man, struggling to make ends meet.
    b. We can't make unilateral decisions just based on the risks posed by the coronavirus. Consider the number of lives that will be lost because of the economic slowdown and its long-term impact.
    c. We need to reopen the economy without putting ourselves in harm's way. The key determinant for that is going to be "Do we have enough resources to protect ourselves and to treat the sick?"

2. **Do Not Throw Caution to the Wind.**
    a. Compared to a month ago, we are more familiar with the situation now. That's good but familiarity breeds complacency, even when the situation is dangerous.
    b. Let's say you are skiing. Just because you are familiar with it, it doesn't mean you ski with flailing arms, right? You maintain caution; that's how you come out safe.
    c. We have built the habit of being cautious over the past month and let's use that habit to our advantage until the danger passes completely.
    d. It's like going on an African expedition. You know there are lions out there, and you've got to protect yourself. Stay inside the van, windows rolled up, and enjoy the safari. Don't do anything stupid.

3. **Be Guided by Your Wisdom.**
    a. We will never have total certainty on when exactly we can reopen the economy. We need to make the best decision using the information at hand. Isn't this the same dilemma we face in other life situations?
    b. There are times when all the information in the world will not guarantee that you will have the right answers. It's like buying a car...you make all the analysis with five spreadsheets and still get the wrong car. Overanalyzing never helps.

   c. Instead, feel from within what's the right thing to do. See what your inner wisdom, your intuition, your common sense is saying. When your intellect doesn't have enough information, you need to use your intuitive wisdom to make decisions. Intuition knows things that intellect doesn't. For that, you need to maintain a calm mind and pay attention to what you feel within.

4. **Individualize Your Decision.**
   a. The decision to embrace the decision to reopen the economy is an individual one. The answer is not the same for everyone. You've got to do what you think is best for you and your loved ones.
   b. If you are still afraid but have enough financial reserves, stay home until the danger passes.
   c. If you are not afraid, when the lockdown is lifted you may go out, but I wouldn't recommend overdoing it. Keep your outdoor activities to the minimum for the time being.
   d. But if you don't have money to feed yourself and your kids, you've got to go out and make money to survive. Again, take all the precautions you can. Act as if the coronavirus is still out there. Don't be afraid but be cautious.

5. **Government Should Step Up.** The government, at the local, state, and national levels, must help people maintain their safety while they go out to restart the economy. Mandates should be passed that everyone must follow some basic rules until the pandemic passes completely:
   a. Every place should have masks and sanitizers. Everyone must maintain social distancing.
   b. Open the economy in phases. Test the waters first. See how things are going. Adjust your approach. Have a taskforce at every level that constantly monitors the situation.
   c. Encourage work from home where possible.

d. More tests should be available for people in every nook and corner of the country. Contact tracing must be done. Quarantine if needed.

e. Antibody tests can help us know if you are already infected and if you are immune to the virus (at least for now).

f. There is no reason why we can't do all this if countries like South Korea and Germany are doing it. We need to learn from and follow the best practices that are already out there.

g. Otherwise, reopening the economy haphazardly may lead to a resurgence of the pandemic, now with vengeance.

Chapter 15:
Coronavirus and Your Immunity

Our greatest weapon against the coronavirus is our immunity. What's immunity? How does it help us fight the virus? What happens inside our body when we are infected with the coronavirus? This is not a medical textbook to go into intricate details and complexities of the immune system. But I will provide you with a helpful overview of how human immunity works and how we can strengthen our immune system to fight this viral infection.

Immunity is your defense system against any foreign organism or particle trying to enter your body. It can be compared to, for example, the United States Armed Forces that is constantly guarding our country and being ever prepared to face any threats from foreign nations. Like we have the Army, Marine Corps, Navy, Air Force, and Coast Guard to meet different needs, in the same way, our immune system is multi-faceted. It deals with different threats in a different way. The immune system is comprised of cells that perform day-to-day general functions as well as highly specialized cells that attack foreign threats in a very precise way. Bone marrow, the spleen, the thymus, and the lymphatic system are the primary places of immune cell production in our body.

I.   **The First Line of Defense:** When a foreign body or a pathogen (bacteria, virus, parasite, or any other harmful microbial organism) tries to enter our body, the first line of defense is our skin and mucus membranes. They offer us a strong barrier against

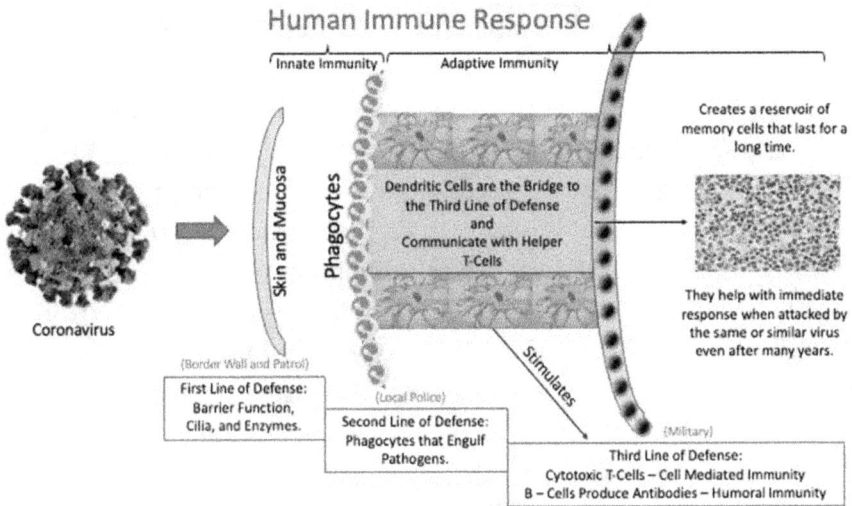

Figure 22

the invasion of foreign bodies. Often, our mucus membranes are lined with cilia (the fine hairlike projections from certain cells such as those in the respiratory tract that sweep in unison and help to sweep away fluids and particles) and also consist of enzymes that dissolve pathogens. We can compare this barrier function of our first line of defense with our border patrol and having a fence or a wall to prevent the invasion of foreigners into our homeland. When that barrier is breached, we get into big trouble. For example, people with skin and mucosal burns are at high risk of death due to infections as the barrier function is lost.

II. **The Second Line of Defense:** If the foreign organisms get past that initial line of defense (often viruses do because they are so minute in size), the second line of defense comes into play in the form of phago- cytic white blood cells. You can compare them to the local police trying to contain the foreign invasion. Phagocytes are those cells that engulf foreign material/organisms and dissolve them. In the case of coronavirus, when someone sneezes, for example, the viral particles gain access to your respiratory tract through the mucus membranes of your nose and then quickly start multiplying by entering your cells. Soon they reach your lungs and continue the multiplication there. Also, these viruses can gain access to your gastrointestinal system through your mouth. The spikes on the coronavirus play a key role in attaching to your cells and then the viral RNA enters your cell, hijacks it totally, and starts making viral proteins that help replicate the virus. It also sends signals to paralyze our immune system.

The phagocytes (our second line of defense, local police) quickly engulf the viruses and try to contain them. But often, the virus multiplies faster than the phagocytes can eliminate them. So, the phagocytes send signals for help. The initial help arrives in the form of "natural killer cells." These are a kind of white blood cells (WBC) that can destroy our own human cells infested with viruses or other pathogens. They send signals to the infected cell to "self-destroy" so that the virus inside the cell dies with it. This is also a part of our second line of defense. While this is being done, a specific kind of phagocyte called "dendritic cell" starts eating up the viral particles, processes them, and presents the "viral antigen" to specialized WBC called lymphocytes to start a more specific immune response against the virus. That is called adaptive immunity, our third line of defense. The first and second line of defense together is called innate immunity, which immediately reacts to foreign threats while a more specific adaptive immunity is underway.

III. **The Third Line of Defense:** The adaptive immunity can be compared to our military system. It is highly specialized and creates a targeted attack against the viruses or any foreign pathogens. A specific type of cell called "helper T-cell" communicates with the "dendritic cell" and takes the "viral antigen" and sends signals to other specialized cells to create a strong response to the viral invasion.

This happens by creating very specific antibodies (by "B-cells") that attach to the viruses and help destroy them and contain the infection. That's called humoral immunity. Also, at the same time, "cell-mediated immunity" is triggered where "cytotoxic T-cells" kill the virus-infested cells. At the same time, "memory B-cells" and "memory T-cells" are generated. Their function is to store in our immune system's memory of the foreign antigen (viruses, bacteria, other microbes) so that when we are again attacked by the same or similar pathogen, our body can react fast and contain the infection.

The communication between various "immune cells" is carried out by a group of proteins called "cytokines," which act as chemical messengers. They help enhance and adapt the immune response according to the nature of the threat.

This in essence is how our immune system works without getting into complex details. It's a simplified version but serves the purpose for now. Now, let's look at the practical implications.

1. **First, we have to appreciate the beauty of our immune system** and how well organized it is in dealing with foreign threats. I can't help but be amazed by its efficiency and effectiveness. Our body does a phenomenal job in protecting us. Without our immune system, we will just die in less than a week.

2. **Do not underestimate your immune system.** It has protected us from various pathogens for thousands of years. It will continue to do so. This specific coronavirus (SARS-CoV-2) is a novel virus that our immune system is still learning about. Our immune system will adapt. It will find a way to protect us. This is particularly important to know from a population health perspective. If this virus is like other coronaviruses—many of them cause the common cold—we should soon find ourselves immune to it, at least for a short while after the exposure and recovery. There is no need to be overly pessimistic about the possibility of a vaccine and proper immune response to the virus.

3. **Would a recovery from COVID protect us from future infections?** No one knows for sure yet. I know our scientists are cautious about whether getting exposed to SARS-CoV-2 will provide us lasting immunity or not. I understand that certain amount of caution needs to be maintained in all scientific endeavors, but my prediction is that we are going to be all right. My educated opinion is that once we develop immunity and antibodies against the virus, it should give us at least short-term protection, for most of us. That is how typically infections work, though there are exceptions. I don't see why this would be an exception if it shares genetics with other coronaviruses.

4. **To support my educated guess, we have some latest research data** from the La Jolla Institute for Immunology. Dr. Alessandro Sette and Dr. Shane Crotty published on May 14 in the online edition

of the journal *Cell* that our body generates a robust immune response to the novel coronavirus, as evidenced by their research in a group of 20 adults who had recovered from COVID-19.

Their Report dispels the theories that the virus may be elusive to our immune system. Though the novel coronavirus (as its name suggests, it's new), it has similarity with other coronaviruses (older versions that cause common cold-like illnesses) to which we get exposed to every year. There is no reason why our immune system can't adapt and fight this virus in time. According to their research, our immune system recognizes the "spike protein" on the virus as well as other viral proteins and elicits good immune response. This is promising as this can pave the path to creating a vaccine sooner than later.

In their own words, "We found that all COVID-19 patients had a solid 'Helper T-cell' response (which helps antibody production) and produced virus-specific 'Killer T-cells', which eliminate virus-infected cells. That means the virus induces what you would expect from a typical, successful antiviral response."

"The teams also looked at the T cell response in blood samples that had been collected between 2015 and 2018, before SARS-CoV-2 started circulating. Many of these individuals had significant T-cell reactivity against SARS-CoV-2, although they had never been exposed to SARS-CoV-2. But everybody has almost certainly seen at least three of the four common cold coronaviruses, which could explain the observed cross reactivity."

These are central findings that can help us win the battle against the coronavirus, and I am proud that I live in the same city, La Jolla, where this research was conducted. I would love to have an opportunity to meet with them once the pandemic is over. Read this article for more information on their research findings: www.lji.org/news-events/news/post/first-detailed-analysis-of-immune-response-to-sars-cov-2-bodes-well-for-covid-19-vaccine-development/)

5. **Now, let's talk about herd immunity**. I wouldn't risk my life, or any one of your lives, on herd immunity. You attain herd immunity when a large group (70% in this case) of people in the community

are immune to the virus, either through recovery from the infection or through vaccination. But whose lives are we going to put at risk, considering that we don't have a vaccine yet? Some are saying it is okay to promote mixing of the people together and develop herd immunity because just the old people die. I am sorry but that's nonsense. Aren't these old people our parents and grandparents? I would fight for them until my last breath. I have personally seen a lot of young people in their 40s and 50s affected badly by this virus. Also, it can attack infants who still have not developed immunity. Whose children are we going to sacrifice? My answer is absolutely no for attaining herd immunity through infection. Every life is important, and we need to protect everyone to the best of our ability. Or else, we are not fit to call ourselves human beings. So, we got to wait until the vaccine is created before we achieve herd immunity. Until then, we must take precaution and common-sense measures while carrying on our daily activities.

6. **What about vaccination then?** I am an eternal optimist. In the past, we have created vaccines that brought terrible diseases like polio, smallpox, measles, mumps, and rubella under control. Some of them were eradicated too! I am positive that we will be able to create a vaccine for SARS-CoV-2 also.

    The ongoing research is promising. The viral "spike protein" could be a target for vaccination as well as some other viral proteins as per the research conducted by Dr. Alessandro Sette and Dr. Shane Crotty at the La Jolla Institute for Immunology, as mentioned above.

    "A single dose of ChAdOx1 nCoV-19, an investigational vaccine against SARS-CoV-2, has protected six rhesus macaques from pneumonia caused by the virus, according to National Institutes of Health scientists and University of Oxford collaborators."

    See this article for details: www.nih.gov/news-events/news-releases/investigational-chadox1-ncov-19-vaccine-protects-mo-nys-against-covid-19-pneumonia

Of course, all this is preliminary research but the direction we are taking is inspiring optimism. It may take a year before we get the vaccine ready for use in humans, but that's not too far from now.

7. **What can we do to boost our immunity?** I wish I can suggest a magic pill that boosts your immunity. There is no scientific evidence that any of the immune boosters sold over the counter are helpful to boost our immunity. The only way to strengthen our immune system is by being nice to it, and that's by adopting a healthy lifestyle. Our body knows what to do and how to protect us, if we take care of it well. Here are some tips:

  i. Sleep well. I mean, have a good, restorative, peaceful sleep. Sleep is one of the greatest healers of our mind and body. I see all the time that people who are low on sleep catch infections or develop autoimmune problems. https://www.hindawi.com/journals/jir/2015/678164/

  ii. Keep stress at bay. Stress is shown to degrade your immune system and make you prone to a variety of illnesses. Keep calm. Be happy. Make it a priority to get rid of stress from your life. https://www.ncbi.nlm.nih.gov/pmc/articles/PMC4465119/

  iii. Eat well, meaning nutritious food. Include lots of fruits, vegetables, and nuts in your diet. They provide vitamins, minerals, and antioxidants that aid in boosting your immunity and living a healthy life. https://www.ncbi.nlm.nih.gov/pmc/articles/PMC6723551/

  iv. Avoid alcohol, drugs, and smoking. Every now and then a drink is okay but don't make it a regular habit. All these substances are known to dampen our immune response and pose dangers to our health. https://www.ncbi.nlm.nih.gov/pmc/articles/PMC5352117/ https://www.ncbi.nlm.nih.gov/pmc/articles/PMC4590612/

  v. Exercise regularly. There is nothing like exercise to keep your body and mind healthy. You don't have to overdo it. But at least 20–30 minutes for 3–4 times a week is bare minimum.

Include aerobic exercises like yoga and stretching in your regimen. https://www.sciencedirect.com/science/article/pii/S2095254618301005

vi. Maintain healthy relationships. Be kind to others. Have some humor. A good smile goes a long way in boosting our immune system and keeping "stress hormones" low. https://www.psychologytoday.com/us/blog/the-happiness-doctor/201706/happiness-and-your-immune-system

Chapter 16:
Living With Corona

Lot has changed in the past few months. We never thought so much change could happen in such a short time. Life will never be the same. There will be a huge shift in our lifestyle at least for the next one year, if not for longer. With no vaccine available yet, we need to continue to take utmost precaution. The good news is that some treatments are available now, though in trial stage, and patient outcomes are promising with medications like Remdesivir, Immune Globulin infusions, convalescent serum, and Interferon alpha-2b. Of course, much larger studies have to be conducted for more definitive guidelines on treatment of COVID-19. I am confident in our scientists, doctors, and researchers that they will find a safe and efficacious treatment available for us soon.

I don't want you to live in fear for the rest of your life. We need to move on and get back to our daily activities as much as we can, sooner or later. That doesn't mean we are going to be reckless and expose ourselves and others to the virus. Do all you want to but by taking good precaution. Here are some final recommendations before we wrap up this book:

I.   **Advice About Media Sensationalism:**
    i.   Take all media reporting with a pinch of salt.
    ii. Remember that even though media is reporting the deaths and disasters caused by the coronavirus, probably it is not applicable to you and the town you live in.

   iii. So, don't be pulled into the negativity created by the news channels. For example, just because thousands of people died in New York, the same is not necessarily true for a town in the Midwest.

   iv. What's happening globally may not happen locally. Respond to the pandemic based on what's going on in your town. Do not live in fear constantly.

2. **Discuss Goals of Care and Advance Directives:**

    i. We must take all the necessary precautions to prevent coronavirus from affecting us, but we should also be prepared for the worse. This is especially true for the elderly with medical problems that increase their risk to have severe illness due to coronavirus.

   ii. If that's the case, you must take the initiative to have your goals of care and advance directives to be written and made clear to your family members so they can make decisions on your behalf, if it comes to that.

  iii. As a physician, I see a lot of patients who are elderly but do not have advance directives when they see me. Sometimes they come with severe illness and they are not in a mental state of making any decisions about their medical care. It puts the family in a dilemma regarding the decisions they must make. This can inadvertently prolong the suffering for the patient.

   iv. So, I urge you to take time to discuss the goals of care and advance directives definitely if you consider yourself at a higher risk of getting severely ill.

    v. There are a few things you need to think about in making these decisions. If you get really ill, do you want to be resuscitated or not? What that means is:

       a. If your heart stops, do you want to get chest compressions?

       b. Do you want to be shocked using a defibrillator, if necessary?

       c. If you can't breathe, do you want to be put on a ventilator/breathing machine?

     d. That often includes intubation, which means having a tube down your trachea/windpipe so that you can be connected to the breathing machine.

     e. People in such situations have to be sedated. You may have to be on the ventilator for many days to weeks if necessary.

     f. Sometimes, if your blood pressure drops, doctors use medications to improve your blood pressure and keep you medically stable.

     g. You also will need to think about having a feeding tube if needed. Usually, this happens when you remain unconscious for a long time or if you have swallowing problems.

  vi. Some people do not want to be resuscitated but some would like to be. Some don't want a feeding tube, but others are okay with it. There is no *one right answer*. Every person is different, and every situation is different. There are a lot of online resources that discuss this topic in detail if you would like to know more.

  vii. I suggest that you take the time to familiarize yourself with these details. If needed, you should contact your physician or an expert who could help you make the right decision.

3. **Prepare a Living Will and Do Some Financial Planning:** This is definitely not my forte, but it would be worth it for you to seek expert advice on it. Be aware of phishing, conning, and financial traps during these chaotic times. If you see anything suspicious, do not share your personal or financial information.

4. **Advice for the Elderly:**

  i. I know it has been difficult for everyone but for you it's even more difficult because of the higher risk of getting severely ill.

  ii. Another issue could be the feeling of loneliness because of self-isolation. The normal social activities are totally cut down. If you have no access to internet or phone, that could pose extra risk for getting socially isolated and getting depressed.

iii. On top of it, the financial impact on you could also be very significant, especially if your savings are invested in the stock market.

iv. During these challenging times, I am sure your friends and family can come to your aid, and you could repay them back later.

v. The key is to use our resources judiciously. Take from others only to have your basic needs met. If your basic needs are met, then be patient until the pandemic passes.

vi. The stock market will recover, and you will recuperate your losses. The economy will bounce back and you will find money again in your pockets.

vii. Please do not imagine the worst possible future. Future is just a figment of your imagination. It's not here yet. Many times, the worst possible future we imagine never comes to pass. Then why add extra stress to our lives?

viii. Stay present. Take one day at a time. Take one moment at a time. Remember, we don't take any money when we leave this world. Don't give yourself a heart attack worrying about money. Focus on your health and mental well-being.

ix. Of course, money is necessary to meet our needs, including medications if we are ill. Just stay put. You will make money again.

x. Rich are those who never lose hope and who remain resourceful even during trying circumstances. A man with a scarcity mentality remains poor even when he is surrounded with riches.

5. **Advice for Youngsters and the Middle-aged:**

i. The youngsters and middle-aged people are the most fortunate during this pandemic. You are getting a lifetime experience of how to respond to a crisis.

ii. The good thing is, the pandemic affects you less than someone who is of advanced age, but that doesn't mean you should throw caution to the wind.

iii. Just because you don't have symptoms doesn't mean you are not infected with coronavirus.

iv. A majority of people have minimal or no symptoms. That means you can be silently carrying the virus and spreading it around, especially to your family members and friends, who may be more vulnerable than you.

v. So, don't be heroic by going out without taking precaution. In fact, taking precaution and being patient until the pandemic passes is the real heroism in this context.

vi. I know probably you are either out of work, working from home, or having many other responsibilities surrounding you during these tumultuous times.

vii. Don't take the difficulties you are facing now too seriously. You have a lot of life ahead.

viii. Do your best each day to further your goals. Take time to reflect upon your life. Reset your goals and objectives.

ix. Put your thoughts on paper. Writing a diary is a good exercise to clear up your mind.

x. Use your time wisely to spend with family. Help others if you can.

6. **Advice for Parents:**

i. The latest reports from New York, Boston, and some European cities are saying now that children are being affected by the coronavirus.

ii. Some children are developing severe disease, causing them to have inflammation throughout their body, which can lead to frighteningly low blood pressure and even death.

iii. This is a relatively new phenomenon that doctors are noticing now that was not observed at the beginning of the pandemic. It seems these could be some late effects of the virus on children after 4–6 weeks of infection.

iv. More data needs to come out on this, but this seems to be a relatively rare phenomenon.

v. It is also possible that the virus is mutating and is changing the way it infects the population as well as which age group it affects.

vi. We still don't know yet what else this virus can do. That's the reason it's called the "novel" coronavirus. Novel means new. When there is a new enemy and we don't know much about it, it's better to be overcautious than undercautious.

vii. So, with children, make sure they are taking all the precautions as you are. I personally would do everything in my capacity to protect my children from this virus. I am sure you would too.

7. **Advice for Health Care Providers:**

i. Me being a doctor at the frontline gave me a direct experience on how to handle the COVID situation. During this pandemic, my respect for my colleagues has multiplied by a thousand-fold.

ii. Each day as I saw the doctors, nurses, emergency responders, physical therapists, nursing aides, and other health care workers putting their lives at risk to help people, I realized how noble our profession is.

iii. Essentially, we are willing to sacrifice our lives for others. That's huge! Not only that, our families are at risk because we interact with so many people and we don't know always for sure who is infected and who is not.

iv. We are afraid that we may carry the virus to our family members. That causes a lot of stress for health care providers. My kudos to all of them at the frontline!

v. My advice for my colleagues is to do your best to protect yourself. Take extra precaution. People who are noble and perform good deeds will get the same favor in return.

vi. The "Law of Karma" is powerful and it never fails. You will be rewarded for your work in one way or another. Good actions never go in vain, though you may not immediately see the results.

vii. I know many of us may be feeling compassion fatigue during this crisis. This is especially true for my global colleagues in big cities like New York.

viii. In New York, doctors saw hundreds of patients dying in front of their eyes, and they were watching helplessly. That can be very traumatic to us. We are meant to save people's lives, not watch them die helplessly.

ix. For those who are traumatized by such experiences, it can be very draining emotionally. Take rest. Take care of yourselves too.

x. Remember, you have done your best. And sometimes that's all we can do. Do not blame yourself for what's happening. There are certain things that are beyond our control. We need to observe the serenity prayer in such instances.

God, grant me the serenity
to accept the things I cannot change,
the courage to change the things I can,
and the wisdom to know the difference.

www.ingramcontent.com/pod-product-compliance
Lightning Source LLC
Chambersburg PA
CBHW050543280326
41933CB00011B/1696